"Practical, insightful, and joyous, *Growing Joy* is a much-needed invitation to renew our relationship with nature—and ourselves—while finding peace in the process."

—Prof. & Dr. Qing Li of Nippon Medical School,
author of *Forest Bathing*

"Filled with tips and thoughtful practices to help us connect to nature and ourselves; *Growing Joy* will not only lead you to take better care of yourself, but of your plants as well, while finding joy in the journey."

—Danae Horst, founder of Folia Collective
and author of *Houseplants for All*

"*Growing Joy* is the breath of fresh air every entrepreneur needs, from greening up your work space to using plants as a tool to disconnect with screens and reconnect with yourself. Failla has a fresh take on how we can use plants to bring more calm to our day-to-day lives."

—Pat Flynn, CEO of Flynndustries and host of
the *Smart Passive Income Podcast*

"*Growing Joy* inspires you to dig deep into the emotional side of making meaningful botanical connections and cultivating a more peaceful lifestyle through plants. As always, Maria offers up a sunny dose of planty joy!"

—Leslie F. Halleck, CPH, author of *Gardening Under Lights, Plant Parenting,* and *Tiny Plants*

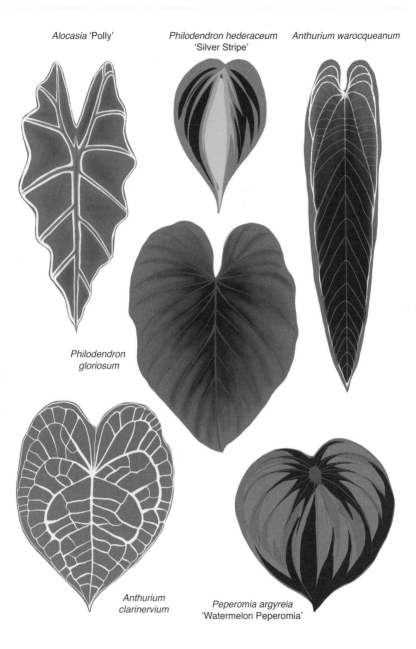

Alocasia 'Polly'

Philodendron hederaceum 'Silver Stripe'

Anthurium warocqueanum

Philodendron gloriosum

Anthurium clarinervium

Peperomia argyreia 'Watermelon Peperomia'

Growing Joy

The Plant Lover's Guide
to Cultivating Happiness
(and Plants)

Maria Failla

Illustrated by Samantha Leung

ST. MARTIN'S
ESSENTIALS
NEW YORK

First published in the United States by St. Martin's Essentials, an imprint of St. Martin's Publishing Group

GROWING JOY: THE PLANT LOVER'S GUIDE TO CULTIVATING HAPPINESS (AND PLANTS). Copyright © 2022 by Maria Failla. Illustrations Copyright © 2022 by Samantha Leung. All rights reserved. Printed in Turkey. For information, address St. Martin's Publishing Group, 120 Broadway, New York, NY 10271.

www.stmartins.com

Designed by Steven Seighman

The Library of Congress Cataloging-in-Publication Data
is available upon request.

ISBN 978-1-250-81489-0 (trade paperback)
ISBN 978-1-250-81490-6 (ebook)

Our books may be purchased in bulk for promotional, educational, or business use. Please contact your local bookseller or the Macmillan Corporate and Premium Sales Department at 1-800-221-7945, extension 5442, or by email at MacmillanSpecialMarkets@macmillan.com.

First Edition: 2022

10 9 8 7 6 5 4 3 2 1

"Gardening:
good for your mind,
good for your
heart, and good
for your ass."

–my mom, Sandy Failla

For my mom,
who taught me how to grow:
in the earth, in my head,
and in my heart.

Contents

A Note from the Author

We've only just met, but I'm going to confess something to you. I wrote this book about joy in what seemed to be the *least* joyful period of my life. Funny how that happens. When I first envisioned this book, I had my list of ideas and practices all lined up and tied in a pretty bow for you. I had been using these tools for years and knew these stories and suggestions would help you disconnect from screens, reconnect with yourself, and blow your freaking mind with moments of awe, peace, and delight. The practices we'll talk about in the coming pages have done exactly that for me and many members of my planty community for many years.

But then there was a little plot twist . . . when the time came around for me to actually *write* this book, my life kind of imploded in the midst of the coronavirus pandemic: I lost my job, my wedding was postponed due to social distancing mandates, and through a series of unexpected events, my partner and I had to move three times within *one* year, with a six-month stint living with my parents—the ultimate romantic dream for any engaged couple. It felt like everything I knew was flipped upside down, and the fear, uncertainty, and loss were all-consuming.

Months into this transitional time, I looked around at my plant collection and noticed that my plants looked miserable: limp leaves, thirsty, yearning for light. Seeing them so unhappy made me pause and realize how much I related to them. In the midst of moving, pivoting, and mourning, I had let the beautiful practices and routines I had developed around my plant collection lapse. This realization hit me like a two-ton bag of potting mix. And then a deeper realization set in: while I let my plant care routine lapse, I had also let my therapy and workout appointments slip through the cracks. I had stopped checking in with friends and my screen time was at an all-time high. My plants and I both needed some serious nurturing.

In that moment, I knew it was time to double down, and "walk the walk" of using plants as not only a tool for joy and self-development, but as a lifeline. I committed to engaging with a plant once a day, every day, and reintroducing these tried and true strategies into my new life circumstances. Ultimately these growing joy practices were stress-tested by the realities of life during one of the hardest seasons I've ever experienced.

Slowly but surely my plants perked up. Slowly but surely, I felt myself coming alive again alongside them. This year, a truth I had known for a while grew deeper roots within me: plant care is an opportunity for self-care.

Growing Joy isn't about the actual plants we cultivate. It's about the feelings that result from witnessing life from a new perspective. It's not *only* about celebrating new growth and blooms, but also about honoring and trusting the dormancy and "lost leaves of our lives." It's about honoring the seasons our plants and we go through, and trusting they are cyclical and will return when it's time. When we can root ourselves in that perspective, anything is possible.

I've written this book about joy, not because it comes easily, but because I've had seasons where I've struggled to find it, and plants have been the answer to my search. Like our plants, joy ebbs and flows, grows and dies back. It shape-shifts, it evolves; it's sometimes easy to find, and sometimes rather elusive. Regardless, we all need more of it in our lives. I don't claim to have all the answers, but I *do* know that if you're open to it—this stuff works. No matter what season of life you are in—whether you are simply looking for some fun ways to enliven your days, suggestions for how to take the next step in plant parenthood, or maybe you're looking for something deeper—wherever you are, I see you, and I'm here for you. Let's grow some joy together, one leaf at a time.

Introduction

It's Growing Season, Baby

I've spent the last several years shouting plants' praises from every mountaintop or microphone I can get to and even made a business around helping people successfully care for plants and cultivate more joy in their lives, but guess what: I used to be an *epic* plant killer. Yep, you heard me right. I, Maria, the author of this book, who've dedicated my life to helping people care for plants . . . have the longest plant-killer criminal record of almost anyone I know. In my plant-killer days, nothing was safe in my home. Although I came from a lineage of incredibly talented Italian farmers and gardeners . . . the gene just seemed to have skipped me.

The cycle would begin with me bringing home the prettiest-looking plant at the grocery store, hoping it would make my home look like an artfully styled Instagram or

Pinterest photo. I treated the plant like another piece of life-less décor and guiltily watched the poor innocent thing die a slow, pathetic death. After my twentieth dead houseplant, I gave up. I labeled myself a "plant killer" and decided to stick with cut flowers instead.

I also used to have little to no relationship with myself. Juggling several minimum-wage jobs to support my career as an actress, and incessantly dieting and beating myself up over my dress size, left very little room for inner work or self-love. Comparing my bank account and career with those of others distracted me from having a loving relationship with myself. Taking pride in how I hustled and "pounded the pavement" took priority over having actual pride or contentment.

To put it simply: When I learned to care for plants, I learned to care for myself. Plants became my greatest teacher. Tightly wound monstera leaves taught me patience, taking days to unfurl the tender, bright green leaves I anxiously wanted to open. My African violet's spontaneous blooms coached me in the art of surprise and delight. My resilient garden showed me how to weather a storm. My first pothos plant, which refused to die, no matter how incorrectly I cared for it, modeled forgiveness. My mother's six-foot-tall sunflowers tutored me in the practice of blooming unapologetically.

Vintage houseplant-care books from the '60s, filled with sage advice, connected me to mentors from a generation

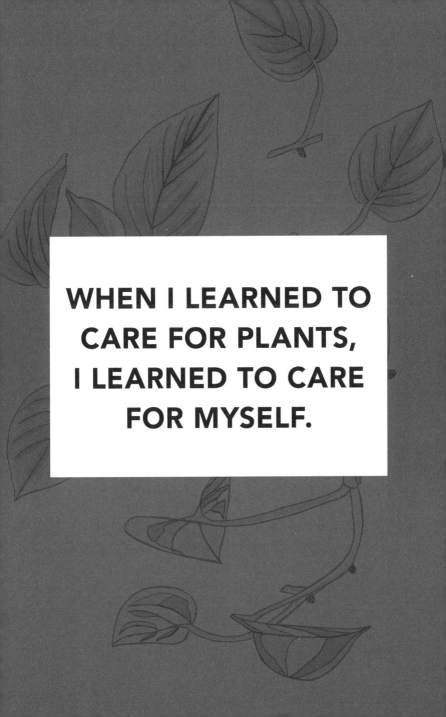

WHEN I LEARNED TO CARE FOR PLANTS, I LEARNED TO CARE FOR MYSELF.

I'll never know. My heartleaf philodendron's slow, consistent, almost unnoticeable growth inspired hope when I felt stuck and unable to move. The strawberries on my balcony reminded me of the importance of dormancy and loss with their promise of more blooms in the coming year. Seeds germinating and thrusting forth their brave cotyledon filled my heart with anticipation and joy.

In my plant-killer days, I had little appreciation for or understanding of the fact that plants were *living* things. I didn't grasp the awesome truth that we had many similarities. These plants, like me, had DNA, were made of thousands of cells, and had the ability to breathe and grow. Most important, they had a fragile life, like mine, that would be lost if uncared for.

I view those "plant-killer years" as a season of dormancy; I was unaware of what I was missing, unaware of the innate part of myself that was longing to connect with nature the way previous generations had.

Learning to care for plants helped me reclaim my right to be connected with nature and wholly alive—existing with the earth, instead of against it. Plants helped me grow into a fuller, more vibrant, more aware version of myself. The joy I received from nurturing them helped me be kinder to myself. As I cared for my plants, moments of connection, empowerment, and joy I never knew were available to me, unfurled.

In this book, I'll share with you the simple practices

and stories from my journey to "Happy Plant Lady," in hopes that you, too, are awakened and develop a lifelong relationship with plants that keeps you curious, joyful, and thriving.

It's growing season, baby.

70% SELF-CARE

20% PLANT CARE

+ 10% STORIES

100% PLANT PUNS

(THE ONLY MATH WE WILL
BE DOING TOGETHER)

How This Book Works

I like to say this book is *part self-care, part plant care, part memoir, and mostly plant puns.* As we travel through this journey together, I'll share a combo platter of simple practices to deepen your relationships with plants and yourself, along with a side of the personal experiences that inspired them.

There's no rocket science or fancy talk here, just simple practices that bring you out of your head, into the present, and toward a more connected, intentional life. I'm going to be real with you . . . some of these practices are silly. Some might feel a little too simple or cheesy. Maintain an open mind, try everything once, and then keep what works and leave what doesn't. I'm on this journey with you, so let's grow some joy together and not take ourselves too seriously.

Things to bring along on this journey to grow joy:

- An open heart and mind
- A journal, to expand on the writing prompts scattered throughout these practices
- A plant or two (one or two is enough; if you are a plant newbie, don't get ahead of yourself—start small and slowly and intentionally grow your collection)
- A dedicated window of time throughout your day to devote to the practices you'll learn in this book. It can be as little as five minutes. We'll discuss this further in Chapter 1.
- Snacks

Throughout the book, you'll find sections called "Dig Deep." These are invitations to think about how lessons you see in nature and in plant care can offer insight into your own growth and development. This is where the magic really happens. Where we get to be more mindful with our approach to our daily lives. I can wax poetic about my experiences, but it's the lessons *you* learn that will grow your own joy. Keep a journal nearby, or schedule some time to return to the book to explore the prompts and reflect. Don't judge your responses; just let the words flow and explore what bubbles up.

So this whole book isn't just me babbling about how cool I think plants are, there will be some interesting concepts and research about the plant/person connection. I'm no scientist, so if you want to nerd out and dive deeper, there are additional science-based resources in the back of this book. Also . . . these nerdy topics and concepts *kill* at parties as conversational tidbits.

At the end of the book you'll also find my "Plant Killer to Plant Person Crash Course." It's an overview of plant care basics inspired by the plant fails I experienced when I was first starting to care for plants. For you newbies, it's a great starter guide to help you feel more confident as you bring new green friends into your home.

This book is really like a delicious buffet: a little of this, a little of that, some sweet, some salty, all set out in front of you in hopes you'll find at least one thing to nibble on that lights you up and helps you grow.

Let's grow some joy, shall we?

Open Your Eyes

Remember in the '90s when all romantic comedies had the female romantic lead who was nerdy and wore glasses, and the male romantic lead who never "saw" her until she took her glasses off, and once she did, all of a sudden he realized that she was beautiful and he'd been in love with her all along and they lived happily ever after? In the story of my life, plants are the beautiful, smart, vibrant, multidimensional woman I was too much of a knucklehead to notice. Once I started successfully caring for plants, and leaning into the joys of plant parenthood, I woke up in sheer amazement to the fact that plants are freaking awesome.

Suddenly, I couldn't *stop* seeing plants. I became acutely aware of the beautiful houseplants that had been in the stores I had been going to for years, but had gone unnoticed. I became captivated by the trees on my street, in awe of their resiliency and ability to thrive in tiny squares of earth in the midst of the concrete sidewalk. I had walked by those trees for years and never noticed them! It was like all the plants I'd never noticed had taken their figurative glasses off and were suddenly right in front of me, waiting for me to finally snap out of my ignorance.

There's a name for this inability to notice the plants surrounding us: plant blindness.

Botanists James H. Wandersee and Elisabeth E. Schussler define plant blindness as "the inability to see or notice the plants in one's own environment—leading to:

a. The inability to recognize the importance of plants in the biosphere, and in human affairs

b. The inability to appreciate the aesthetic and unique biological features of the life-forms belonging to the plant kingdom; and

c. the misguided, anthropocentric ranking of plants as inferior to animals, leading to the

erroneous conclusion that they are unworthy
of human consideration."[1]

We don't notice plants, therefore we can't value them. If we can't notice and appreciate the plants in our offices, on our block, or in our neighboring forests and parks, how can we effectively appreciate and care for our sweet planet?

Plant blindness is a powerful concept and one that will frame our journey in *Growing Joy*, but it is important to acknowledge that the way we become desensitized to the plants and nature around us doesn't compare with or diminish the experience of those who experience physical blindness. In her book *Lessons from Plants*, Beronda Montgomery suggests the use of "plant bias" instead, which is how we will refer to this concept moving forward.

Wandersee and Schussler also talk about the importance of having a "plant mentor," a "knowledgeable and friendly" guide to help highlight the wonderful world of plants and awaken young people out of plant bias. I've been told I'm knowledgeable. I've also been told I'm friendly. I will talk about my obsession with plants and the lessons they've taught me till I'm blue in the face. I'd love to help. Although . . . "plant mentor" feels too lofty for me, so I'll stick with the term "plant friend."

Wanna be plant friends?

Rooted in Routine

There's a quiet, planty revolution happening in homes around the world. People from all walks of life, in all corners of the world, are letting plants and the act of caring for them peel back their layers of overwhelm, overstimulation, and unwillingness to be with their own thoughts. They're finding that plants reveal moments of awe, presence, and joy that are rocking their worlds.

Caring for plants is about bringing life into your home, watching it unfold before your eyes, and being a part of its success or failure. This is a life-long hobby. Our plant collections have so much to share with us, but **we have to make time to listen**. We make that time by creating a routine around our plant care practices. But here's the kicker, our plant care routines aren't only for our plants. This time is also for us—to disconnect from screens and the hustle and bustle of life and find a moment of connection and reflection.

When you set an intention to show up for yourself in a particular way, and follow through, you build confidence and feel empowered. Setting up a structured routine around your plant care practice helps tune you to the frequency of their growth and warns you when something might be going wrong. Seeing the entire life cycle of a flower or new leaf unfurl is a practice of patience and commitment. Consistency helps deepen your connection with your plants and creates space and time for you to open up to the lessons they're waiting to teach you.

Start a plant care routine, show up, and become your plants'—and your own—best caretaker.

Look at a Plant Before You Look at a Screen

If you take anything away from this book, please let it be this: This simple and intentional practice has created more stillness and joy in my life than any expensive yoga retreat I've been to, workout class I've taken, or self-help book I've read (and I've read them all). It's truly this simple: Look at a plant before you look at a screen when you wake up. In fact, look at several! Spend as much time as possible interacting with your plants in the morning before your screen-time adventures begin.

I used to live for the "hack" of using my phone to wake up faster in the morning, because the blue light from the screen jolts your brain out of its natural, slower "power up" mode. I'd essentially start my day by giving up my agency:

allowing external factors like email, texts, and triggering social media posts and videos to dictate how the rest of my day would play out. It was a lovely distraction from my own thoughts when I did not want to be alone with them. This seemingly benign habit put me in a reactive state the rest of the day. It gave me no time to reflect on what was going on, plan for what I wanted to accomplish, or think about how I wanted to show up for myself and the world that day.

Once I started my balcony garden, things changed. I started finding so much happiness in the slow, luxurious time spent with my plants. Sitting there, with my journal, I'd dream about my long-term goals, write my gratitude list, and just sit with myself and see what thoughts bubbled up.

Looking at a plant before a screen to start my day allowed for true "me time," for listening to my inner voice and having a little dialogue with her. It was the first time in a long time (maybe ever) that I had actually been still with myself and my thoughts. I finally gave myself permission to simply clear my mind and "be." This practice gave me a moment of stillness amidst the insanity that is living in New York City.

Looking at a plant before you look at a screen—which really means engaging with yourself before engaging with the world—is like *putting armor on to prepare for whatever the day throws at you.* Spend time with plants before you lose yourself to technology, your calendar, or other people's problems. It's a simple shift that will change your life.

Can you armor up, plant friend?

Strategies to Look at a Plant Before You Look at a Screen

Break up with your morning cell phone routine

Growing Joy is about reclaiming time with yourself through plant care, but in order to reclaim that connection with ourselves, we must rework the habits that have gotten us to the numb, disconnected state we're in. Getting a quick hit of screen time in the morning can be as addictive as the first cup of coffee to start your day. But it's time to break this bad habit and to allow the magic to unfold before your eyes.

This is easier said than done. Smartphones, with their built-in alarms, text messages, email notifications, and social media apps, have made it extremely difficult to operate without them. So let's set some ground rules to break the sneaky habit of letting your phone run your life:

- Sleep with your phone in a different room. Every night I tell my Google Home to wake me up the next day, and it obliges. You could go a step further and use a real old-fashioned alarm clock, and enjoy the retro feel of being truly disconnected from wireless media.

- Commit to not responding to work emails before your official workday starts
- Decide each morning on a nonnegotiable time before which you will remain phone-free
- Utilize the "Do Not Disturb" option most phones have and set windows of time your phone won't interrupt your sleep schedule or morning practice

Be kind to yourself, plant friend. It's *hard* to separate from our phones. Cultivating awareness around this habit is the first step in creating space for reconnecting with yourself. You've got this.

Keep a plant or two by your bed

No outdoor space for a traditional garden? No problem! Just keep a plant or two (or ten) in your bedroom. As you wake up, allow yourself to slowly open your eyes and simply direct your focus onto the plant. Notice the leaves and the way the light filters onto them. Let your mind slowly wake up the way it's designed to.

Breathe. Notice what thoughts are present.

Breathe. Enjoy the absence of thought. Keep breathing

mindfully and don't look at your phone—even if you really, really want to.

I have two Swiss cheese plants *(Monstera deliciosa)* right next to my bed. The heart-shaped leaves cascade over their pots and moss poles and dangle over the bed. When I wake up, it looks like they are waving at me, wishing me a good morning. It's adorable. I've also lined the windowsills of my bedroom with plants so that when I get up, I walk past several more plants before I can even get to my precious coffee.

Wherever your normal foot traffic brings you in the morning—to the coffee machine, bathroom, windows, or couch—figure out how to place plants there and engage with them before you start focusing on technology. It will be tough at first, but it will be completely worth it once you get used to being with yourself again.

Have (screen-free) morning garden time

If you have a balcony or outdoor space, what are you waiting for!? Get out in your garden in the morning and leave your phone inside! A garden with herbs, tomatoes, and vegetables (or just one of the three) will give you plenty of things to do before looking at screens in the morning. Take your pick: watering, weeding, pruning, tidying, or simply enjoying your plants' beauty. Swing by the "Engage Your Senses" chapter for all sorts of fun ways to interact with them. When you start your day in the garden, you'll come back feeling grounded and proud that you've already accomplished something—even before you open your in-box.

If you don't have outdoor space, you can always try growing a small herb or two on a sunny windowsill, in a hydroponic setup, or under grow lights indoors. See the "Grow Your Own Food" section of this book for more on this.

A Snapshot of My Plant-Killer Morning Routine

Chimes drift into my subconscious, getting louder and louder. I rummage for my phone, hit "snooze" for the third time, and roll back over to sneak in another eight minutes of sleep. After a full hour of snoozing (don't judge), my guilt finally triggers me to grab my phone and turn off the alarm, only to begin another unfortunate habit of mine: scrolling. Lying in bed, before my feet even hit the ground, I'll have already checked my Instagram messages, scrolled my Facebook feed, and checked my emails. The blue light of the screen helps drag me out of the morning brain fog. I roll myself out of bed and beeline for the coffee maker.

Coffee time: my phone becomes the companion to my morning coffee routine. More scrolling as I impatiently wait for my Nespresso to pump out my fuel for the day. Another email, ten minutes passing as I watch a YouTube makeup tutorial, another ten lost to a *Say Yes to the Dress* clip. I snap out of the social media warp hole and realize just how late I've managed to make myself. At this point, I turn into a human Tasmanian devil and whirl around my apartment to get ready and rush out the door. I anxiously bounce from appointment to appointment, distract myself with phone calls on my short walks to the subway, binge podcasts on my commute, or memorize lines for my next audition.

In the blink of an eye, the day is over, and I'm cozy on my couch with my partner, Billy, ready for the next Netflix binge. I bookend the day with a little light scrolling on Instagram in bed before the cycle of screens and appointments starts again tomorrow.

A Snapshot of My Plant Lady Morning Routine

Chimes drift into my subconscious, getting louder and louder. I still hit "snooze" most days, because my bed is cozy and the floor is lava. I turn off my alarm and confidently resist the small itch to open any apps. I sleepily turn my attention to the Swiss cheese plant (*M. deliciosa*) sitting next to me on the nightstand. I take a few deep breaths and allow my eyes to slowly, naturally wake up as I notice that a new leaf has grown and is beginning to unfurl.

Breathe in: I notice the prehistoric beauty of the emerald leaves dappled with holes, an entire constellation in a single blade. My eyes drift from the pattern of the holes to slowly trace the leaf's heart-shaped outline.

Breathe out: I watch one sunbeam stream across the entire plant, noticing the shadows it creates. Chiaroscuro: light and dark dancing within such fine lines. A reminder of the lightness and darkness that dances within me. I remind myself to turn the plant's pot, to give every leaf a fair shot at sunshine.

Breathe in: I reach out to wipe some dust that's settled on the surface of the leaf, revealing its delightfully smooth skin, and take a moment to notice the tiny veins running through the blade: a superhighway of paths, varied in size, all working together to help this little plant stand up and thrive. Never stop trying to find your light, little guy.

Breathe out: Coffee time.

Morning coffee now takes place away from my couch and my phone, on my tiny balcony. By "tiny," I mean hilariously tiny. Too tiny to use, really. I perch on a cushion on the doorframe with my coffee, surrounded by my modest balcony garden setup. Steady basil, wacky mint, spicy oregano, slender chives, and an adorable, potted tomato plant whose scent transports me to my *Nonni*'s—my grandmother's—garden. Sun tickles my skin as the symphony of scents brings me into the present. I pinch a basil leaf and notice how potent the smell becomes as I gently crush the leaf between my fingers.

I feel slightly high after a deep inhale of invigorating

rosemary, like the scent is tickling my brain. All of my attention is absorbed by a dewdrop slowly gathering itself before it tumbles from the underside of a basil leaf. It's patience incarnate. It doesn't leave a moment too soon, or stay past when it's welcome. "What is my next big leap? When will I drop?" I wonder.

Thoughts drift in and out of my mind:

I greet them,
I release them,
I breathe.
I drink my coffee.
Space.
Peace.

It's exquisite, and foreign.

In this quiet moment, surrounded by natural light and this lush collection of plants, I find the space between. It is a sacred place: after I wake and before my calendar dictates my day. A space to peel back expectation, pressure, comparison, and all of the other influences of everyday life. A space to ask myself questions and let myself answer them. A space to get to know myself better.

Then the day of appointments begins. The schedule is the same, but the seeds of peace planted during that morning garden moment grow throughout my day. My back-to-back meetings don't feel as overwhelming. The crowded subway rides are less anxiety-ridden. The nightly Netflix binge still happens, but ends earlier. Something is different. I am different—more grounded, more me.

In the winter, this practice moves from my small balcony to my teensy apartment and the windowsills, which are filled with the inviting shapes and colors of my collection of houseplants. Each morning, we visit. We are old friends now. Ride or die. I take time to check in, celebrate their defiant growth, cheer on a timid opening flower bud, make peace with lost leaves, and water when necessary. My feelings and experiences with my plant collection are eerily similar to my feelings and experiences in life. These plants have become my confidants, my green guides in my continual journey to understand myself and the world around me.

Create a Plant Care/Self-Care Routine That Works for You

I understand that not everyone is a morning person, and not everyone will find joy in waking up early to spend time with plants—or waking up early for any reason whatsoever, for that matter. Some people might want to punch me in the face at the mere suggestion of a morning practice. I get it. Kudos to you for understanding your boundaries and limits. The key to growing joy is to establish a routine and stick with it, in order to reap the benefits and the magic of observing continual growth and of tending to a living, changing thing. That can happen at any time of day.

If the idea of creating a routine, regardless of the time of day, sounds nightmarish to you, suck it up and try it anyway! Routines may be hard to create, but they are the freaking best. Remember they build confidence, set you up for success as a plant parent, and create space for you to find all sorts of new joyful moments that are going to rock your socks off. The routine you cultivate will move from a chore to something you look forward to, as you grow alongside your plants and allow more peace and joy in your day.

Choose a recurring time that feels natural to you and simply commit to turning off your computer, setting aside your mental to-do list and the stress of the day, and engaging with your plants. Screen-free time is important here. The frequency and time of day will look different for everyone. We've covered the morning option, but unwinding and hanging with your plants after a busy workday is a great alternative. Others might enjoy a midday pick-me-up, to get away from their desks and computers and realign. Others might set aside time on Sundays to get quiet, connect, and prep for the week to come. Whatever works for you, just stick to it. The time of day doesn't matter, but the frequency and consistency does.

Here are some activities to do in this sacred time:

- Watering (but *only* when your plants need it; check if it's time to water by putting your finger in the soil to feel for dampness, at the same time taking a moment to be present and leaning into the sensation of the soil on your fingertips)

- Wiping dust off leaves

- Inspecting the underside of leaves, soil, and stems for pests and signs of disease

- Rearranging and styling your plants in different ways around your home based on your mood

- Rotating the pots of plants that are leaning toward the light source. Light-responsive hormones in a plant trigger it to stretch its leaves toward a light source to harvest as much light as possible for photosynthesis. This response is called phototropism. If light is too low, especially on one side of the plant, it may lean so far toward the light it can tip over. Rotating your pots allows your plants to remain better balanced and upright. Check the "Understanding Light" section on page 215 for more information about photosynthesis.

- Removing any yellowing or browning leaves
- Trying any of the practices in this book that catch your eye

Note: A plant care routine *does not* equal a watering routine. Many new plant parents often overwater their plants out of their desire to engage with them on a daily basis. It's important to structure your plant care routine so you interact with your plants on a daily or weekly basis, *but* only water your plants when they need to be watered.

Dig Deep

Questions to ask yourself during your plant care routine

There are so many plant/person parallels to learn from, if you look closely. While you incorporate these practices into your daily or weekly routine, ask yourself these questions and see what comes up.

Routine	Questions to ask yourself
Watering your plants (only when they need it!)	How hydrated am I today? Do I need to water myself? What is replenishing me emotionally right now?
Wiping dust off leaves	What areas of my life are feeling stagnant and need a little metaphorical "dusting" off? Take a moment to observe your own emotions—what feelings have been lingering that you might have been avoiding?
Checking moisture levels in the soil	How do you feel in your body in this moment? What might you need more or less of—sleep, food, exercise?
Inspecting the underside of leaves, soil, and stems for pests and signs of disease	What areas of my life have a toxic element I need to address? What routine maintenance and self-care can I be exploring in my own life?
Rotating the pots of plants who are leaning towards their light source	What positive elements of my life can I develop? What am I excited to focus on right now?
Pruning any yellowing or browning leaves	What isn't serving me right now? What can I prune away?

Grow Gratitude

Writing down three things you are grateful for every day is a free, easy way to gift yourself immediate perspective and a boost of confidence in the kick-ass life you've got, but might not recognize. It's so easy to get swept away in the negativity of day-to-day stressors. This simple practice helps you "see the forest for the trees," pulling you out of that daily minutiae and giving you a larger appreciation for your awe-inspiring, miraculous life.

Too often we take the many beautiful gifts in our life for granted: the roof over our head, our partners, our health, our families, even the simple support of the chair we sit on. You're alive and you have air in your lungs—how freaking amazing is that?!! Showing gratitude for the seemingly unimportant things in your day is a wonderful practice in reframing just how freaking awesome the one life we've got to live truly is.

Dig Deep

Find a quiet moment, sit with your plants, and write a gratitude list in your journal; or run through it in your head as a walking meditation when you visit with your plants. It's a beautiful way to start or reset your day and will be an immediate joy booster.

Here are some journaling prompts to get you growing:

- What is bringing you joy right now?
- What areas of your life do you feel confident in?
- When you wake up in the morning or when you start a new week, what do you look forward to?
- Who are you thankful for? Take a deep breath and send those people some loving, positive thoughts.
- What are the top three things you are thankful for today?
- What difficulty have you had in the past that you can be thankful for now?

Grow gratitude. Grow contentment. Grow a big, lush, abundant life as gorgeous as any photo-worthy plant.

Stress: The Joy Killer

Feeling imbalanced? It might have something to do with your autonomic nervous system (ANS). The sympathetic and parasympathetic nervous systems were things I heard a lot about in the self-help books I've read and wellness retreats I've been on, but I never quite understood what they meant. So here's the gist: The ANS is the part of our nervous system responsible for the functions in our body that happen naturally, like breathing, digestion, organ function, and reflexes. It's divided into two branches you've probably heard about: the sympathetic and parasympathetic nervous systems. The responses triggered by these systems are complementary to each other and work alongside each other in harmony to keep us balanced and happy.

The sympathetic nervous system response, nicknamed "fight or flight," ensures our survival. When it kicks in, our adrenaline and circulation increase, our alertness goes through the roof, our sense of smell heightens, and our digestion slows to send blood and resource to our brain and extremities in order to prepare us to fight or flee. It's basically our survival kit for meeting a dangerous situation, like encountering a bear or similar threat, and getting the heck out of there. This is a necessary survival response, and we should be extremely grateful for it.

The parasympathetic response does the opposite. Nicknamed "rest and reset," "rest and digest," or "feed and breed," it helps slow things down, lowers our heart rate, increases blood flow to our reproductive organs and digestive system, and helps with relaxation and restoration. It's what calms us down after the "fight or flight" feeling we've all experienced when we realize we missed a deadline at work or when we find ourselves alone in a subway car at midnight.

Here's the issue: These two systems should work together within the ANS to regulate our bodies, emotions, and wellness. Unfortunately, modern life, with its traffic, money woes, twenty-four-hour news cycle, unending email in-box, and general "go go go" mentality, can kick us into consistent, chronic, "fight or flight" mode and allows for little rest and reset. This imbalance can leave us feeling drained, burned out, and depressed—not a good look on anyone.

Since we're living in that high-anxiety, "fight or flight" mode more often these days, it's important to understand and recognize the imbalance and work to find ways to incorporate more parasympathetic, rest and reset activity in our bodies.

When you need a moment to rest and reset, try "Taking 5" with your plants.

Take 5 and Have a Meditative Moment with Plants

I have a bit of a love/hate relationship with meditation. I've had seasons where I swear by meditation and worship gurus and look forward to my practice every day. I have other seasons in life where I can't bring myself to sit still and clear my mind, even if someone paid me. The formality of what one thinks of as "meditation"—sitting still and allowing for the absence of thought—can be extremely overwhelming to our busy, over-stimulated brains. Once I found my herb garden and plant collection, stillness became much easier. Quiet became more enjoyable. Plants are a sneaky way to practice mindfulness without the intimidating formality of traditional meditation.

GET YOUR OM ON WITH PLANTS

In this practice, the only objective is quiet and stillness. If you associate meditation only with sitting cross-legged on a pillow while chanting, stop. When we "Take 5 with plants" we are simply looking to clear our minds, or at least calm them down. I'm not asking you to become the Dalai Lama, I'm just asking you to bravely step away from distraction and drop in on yourself.

Let's find some clarity and stillness, shall we? The objective is to hang with your plants and be still and quiet for five minutes. Once you get comfortable with five minutes, you can play around with increasing your time, but let's not get ahead of ourselves. Five minutes. It can be as simple as that. You've got this.

Amazing Times to Take 5

- Waking up in the morning before you've engaged with a screen (my favorite way)
- In the midst of a long work session, when your eyes and brain can use a break
- Whenever you catch yourself in or about to go down a worry spiral
- Before you have a big meeting and you want to center yourself
- Before bed as a way to quiet your mind

Steps to enjoying a meditative moment with your plant:

1. Walk over to your favorite plant, or keep one strategically placed in your sight line where you sleep, work, or make your coffee in the morning.

2. Put your hand on your belly button for a moment and focus your attention on the movement of your breath. Take slow breaths, in and out. Hear the air pass through your nose and throat. Close your eyes, drop inward, and be still with yourself for three cycles of breath. *In, 2, 3, 4. Hold, 2, 3, 4. Out, 2, 3, 4. Hold, 2, 3, 4.*

3. Look at your plant and let your mind wander. Meditate on any of these prompts that resonate with you:

   - Observe the shape of the leaves and the patterns of the veins within them.

   - Observe how the leaves grow off the stem: What patterns do they grow in? Are they in little groups? Do they all grow off one side of the stem or in alternating patterns?

   - Trace the shapes of the leaves with your fingers.

   - Notice and feel the texture of the leaves: fuzzy? slick? waxy?

- Notice how light interacts with a leaf. Does it illuminate the leaf as it reflects off a shiny surface? Does it cast shadows on some leaves and not others? Does it shine through the leaf?

- If you are sitting below a plant, look upward toward the light and experience the plant from below. (You can also just pick up a plant and hold it toward a light source.) Notice how different the color, veins, and patterns look from below.

- Look for new growth. Can you see new buds, or leaves unfurling? Watching a new leaf unfurl or flower open over the course of the week is a beautiful opportunity to practice patience and revel in anticipation.

Take 5 with your plants as part of your daily routine, and use this simple practice whenever you wish to check in with yourself, take a breath, pause, and reset.

Pepper these nuggets of stillness throughout your day to give yourself restorative breaks. They are sweet, peaceful moments that will bring you back to yourself and plant seeds of stillness within your soul to grow throughout your day.

The Great
Outdoors

Time for some cold, hard, scary facts. The average American spends around 90 percent of his or her time indoors.[1] Yes, you read that statistic correctly: We spend the majority of our lives indoors, disconnected from the natural surroundings we evolved in, breathing dusty air, fixating on screens, sitting on our couches. How has our society become so far removed from the "go outside and play till sunset" generations before us? The scariest part of this data is that this statistic was published *before* the popularity of Netflix and Chill, Call of Duty, TikTok, and, well, the internet, which has led to even more time behind windows and walls.

Listen, I'm as guilty as they come here. I've had moments when I've realized I haven't left my home in forty-eight hours thanks to the modern conveniences of restaurant delivery, Zoom calls, and Amazon. It's so freaking easy to become part of this statistic. But it's also important to understand the problem, realize the slippery slope of a social media feed and Netflix binge (once again . . . guilty), and actively intervene by taking a daily walk outdoors or spending thirty minutes with your plants and your own original thoughts.

We weren't designed to spend this much time looking at screens and peeking into other people's curated worlds. Although screen addiction isn't a diagnosed disorder yet, it's a clear issue for many who don't remember a time without access to instant internet. Our inability to adapt to the rapid technological advancements even has a name now: technostress.[2] You don't need a million scientific studies to understand that more screen time + packed schedules + social media addiction = anxiety and decreased well-being. I'm sure you've experienced this in your own body at some point—and it's time to make a change.

I know this sounds like a bummer, but there is good news, too: Studies are also proving that exposure to nature can do a myriad of amazing things for our bodies and wellness, such as increase our capacity for empathy, generosity, and trust,[3] help hospital patients recover faster[4] and use fewer painkillers, and even make us happier. The mere presence of trees in urban areas can decrease depression rates[5] and improve your sense of well-being. One study shows that being around nature can make you feel as good as getting a $10,000 raise.[6] Another showed that sitting in nature lowers cortisol (stress hormone) levels by 12 percent and decreases sympathetic nervous activity (fight or flight) by 7 percent.[7] Who doesn't want those fantastic benefits in their life?!

It's time to reconnect with nature, whether it's "the real thing" outdoors or an indoor jungle you create and cultivate from the convenience of your home. An invisible thread ties us to the natural world around us. *We just have to tug a little to remember it.*

Attention Restoration Theory

Attention Restoration Theory, pioneered by husband and wife team Dr. Stephen and Dr. Rachel Kaplan, is a concept I love. It demonstrates the importance of surrounding ourselves with nature. But before we dive in, let me remind you that this is a *theory.* It's an interesting idea to explore in your journey to re-connecting with nature and yourself. So take what you want, leave the rest, and keep reading and digging deeper.

ART revolves around two types of attention: directed and involuntary. Both are crucial to our survival. Directed Attention is all about focus. It's voluntary, requires effort, and is super important for us to use when completing important tasks and learning. With Directed Attention, you block out external stimuli to focus on what you are doing, which is crucial for us to be effective and useful.

But there's a downside—too much repetitive, forced Directed Attention can be taxing. It isn't sustainable and can bring on fatigue. You know when you work really hard on a long project for an extended period of time and at the end you feel "mentally exhausted"?[8] That could be too much Directed Attention at work.

The second type of attention, Involuntary Attention,

also referred to as "Fascination," is effortless and sustainable. It requires a stimulating environment for someone to naturally engage in, like watching clouds pass in the sky, listening to the rustling of leaves, or walking through a forest—you don't need to focus directly on anything, but simply take in your surroundings. The Kaplans say that Involuntary Attention in a restorative environment can help us recover from the fatigue brought on by too much Directed Attention. With all of the delightful distractions and opportunities to use Directed Attention these days, we run the risk of becoming mentally fatigued if we don't find and create more opportunities for the sweet, restorative Involuntary Attention our bodies and minds crave.

We'll dive deeper into how to use concepts in ART in our homes later, but it's interesting to know that multiple studies now show how nature can heal fatigue. Being exposed to a natural scene, even for as little as forty seconds,[9] can help our effectiveness in tasks that require Directed Attention.

More and more research is surfacing that proves the important relationship between connection with nature, our well-being, and the greater good of our planet. Whether it's by engaging with nature on a larger scale with hikes, long walks, or camping, or on a smaller scale by using houseplants to intentionally disconnect from your screens, it's up to us to figure out what our path to reconnection is, follow what feels good, and marvel at what unfolds.

Forest Bathing, aka Get Outside!

How I adore the glorious Japanese art of *Shinrin-yoku*! In Japanese, *shinrin* means "forest" and *yoku* means "bath," so the art of *Shinrin-yoku* is to "take in the forest through your senses," aka bathing your senses in all the forest has to offer. We are not talking about running through your local park with earbuds blasting your favorite podcast while Snapchatting your route; we are talking about intentional, deliberate time spent in the forest, appreciating trees and slowing the heck down. It's amazing—you've got to try it.

Forest Bathing has been part of the Japanese culture and even national health programs since 1982. As I write this book, the Forest Therapy Society offers profiles of sixty-three certified Forest Therapy Bases in Japan. A Forest Therapy Base is described as a forest "where the relaxing effects have been observed based on scientific analysis conducted by a forest medical expert."[10]

I can't talk about Forest Bathing without mentioning Dr. Qing Li, chairman of the Japanese Society for Forest Medicine and my plant nerd crush. Dr. Li has been on the forefront of Forest Therapy research, and his book *Forest Bathing* changed the way I live my day-to-day life. In it, Dr. Li shares study after study proving that Forest Therapy can reduce blood pressure, lower stress, improve cardiovascular and metabolic activity, lower blood sugar levels, improve concentration and

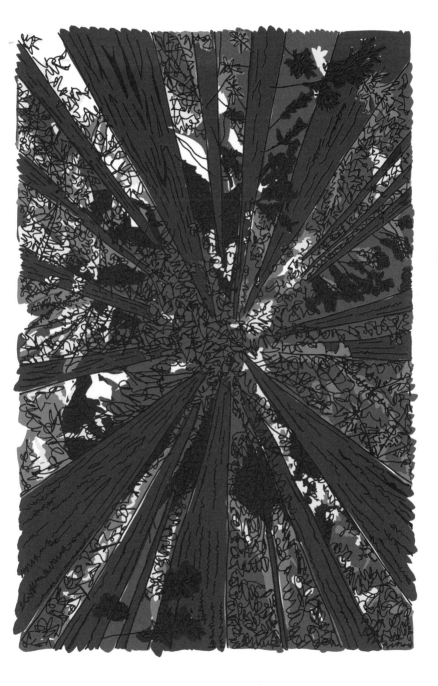

memory, lift depression, improve pain thresholds, improve energy, boost immune systems with an increase in the body's nature killer (NK) cells, and help regulate weight.[11]

Are you sold yet? Ready for some Forest Bathing basics?

Forest Bathing Basics

- Find the closest forest or park near you.

- Leave your phone, camera, headphones, and any other technology behind, or at least turned off in your pocket.

- Go for a walk. Slow your steps and breathing down; allow yourself to stop and admire your surroundings. There's no destination—it's all about the journey.

- Be present. Breathe deeply.

- Engage your five senses: What do you see? What do you hear? How does the forest smell? Can you taste the fresh air? Stroke leaves, feel the soil between your fingers, dip your toes in the river. Follow your instincts. I like to approach different trees and rub their leaves and inhale their scent.

- Notice what feelings rise up. Greet them and release them.

- If you find a nice spot to sit, go for it. This isn't about physical activity as much as about being present in nature and engaging your five senses.

- Count all of the different forest sounds you can hear. How many birds are singing? Is there a babbling brook? Revel in the heady sound of rustling leaves.

- Dr. Li recommends Forest Bathing for two hours if possible, but we can feel the effects in as little as twenty minutes.

Try and make Forest Bathing a habit, not just a onetime thing. It can be as simple as taking your lunch break in a nearby park a few times a week, or as extensive as scheduling monthly camping trips.

Experience trees in whatever capacity you can, and do it on repeat. You won't regret it.

Gentle Giants

We humans think we have everything figured out and that we're so impressive, but we've got nothing on old-growth redwood trees (*Sequoia sempervirens*). These "ever-living redwoods" are living examples of the power of community and adaptation. I had the opportunity to see these gentle giants up close and personal at the Henry Cowell Redwoods

State Park. The tallest tree in the park is 277 feet tall, fifteen feet wide, and around fifteen hundred years old.

Stepping into this park felt like stepping into another world. As I moved from the sunny, hot parking lot into the cool darkness of the forest, I could feel my anxiety drop as much as the temperature did. Entering this magical oasis, I half expected a small fairy to flit over and offer us a tour. The sheer magnitude of the trees was disorienting at first, so unfamiliar that it forced you to second-guess the scale of your entire life. Gaping at them in awe, I realized that these trees were here for over a thousand years before me, and will be around long after I'm gone. They embodied a quiet power that was both invigorating and deeply peaceful. In their presence I instinctively stood taller and breathed deeper.

Did you know that redwood trees have tannins in their bark that give them their signature cinnamon red color and help ward off insects and even fire? Many of them have survived forest fires. Even after being hollowed out by the flames, they've maintained their structure and ability to rebuild their tissue over time. Talk about tenacity! Redwoods have the unique ability to grow new trees from an old trunk base. If a redwood is cut down, its root system typically remains alive and may help a family of new trees grow around the old tree trunk, bringing forth a new generation. Talk about generosity. The resilient roots of a living tree can spread laterally across a forest as wide as the tree is tall, growing around and with the roots of other trees and allowing all of them to stabilize and support each other.[12] Talk about teamwork.

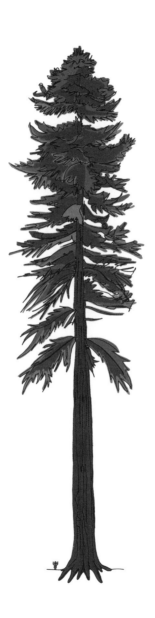

LESSONS LEARNED FROM REDWOOD TREES

Stand up straight and proud.

Slow and steady wins the race.

Keep going, even after something tries to burn you down. You are more resilient than you think.

Grow strong roots, share them with those around you.

Support others.

Your uniqueness is what makes you resilient.

There is power in silence.

Zone Out in a Fractal Pattern

Fractal patterns are one of nature's best-kept design secrets. There are lots of fancy mathematical definitions of fractals, but essentially a fractal is a shape that is made up of mini, almost identical versions of itself. Richard Taylor, a pioneer in fractal research (don't even get me started on his triumphs identifying fractals in Jackson Pollock paintings; look it up—it's a thing), explains it this way: "Fractals consist of patterns that recur on finer and finer scales, building up shapes of immense complexity."

Next time you are outside, notice how the branch from a tree or the frond of a fern (*Polypodiophyta* spp.) is actually a tiny mini-me of the tree or fern as a whole. After learning about this concept, I went for a walk to allow myself ample opportunity for Involuntary Attention and Fascination. But I couldn't take more than two steps without staring in amazement at all the fractals I saw everywhere around me. A large trunk splits into two, which splits into four, then divides into eight, all the way to the teensiest branch. The pattern is so simple up close, but on the large scale of a tree it's impressive.

So next time you take a walk outside or sit with your plant collection, get lost in the spiral of a seashell or the veins of a leaf. Revel in the delicate lace pattern of a snowflake or a fern frond's delicious intricacies.[13–16] Your brain and body will thank you for it.

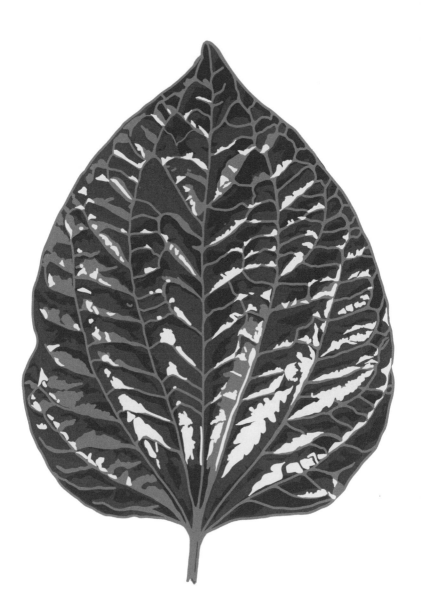

A Dose of Forest Medicine

The 2020 COVID-19 pandemic sucked for most people, and I was not an exception. Before my time as a plant lady podcaster, I had a decade-long career as a musical theater performer. When COVID hit, I was performing in my dream show, at my dream theater in NYC when the social distancing mandates forced my show to close, three days before opening night. The theater industry evaporated in front of my eyes, leaving actors in shock and wondering where the next paycheck would come from. My fully planned wedding was postponed, as we feared that the hugs and dancing we were looking forward to could in fact kill the people we loved most.

On top of those two major setbacks, my partner (then my fiancé) and I temporarily moved back in with my parents for six months. Our period of engagement was the opposite of what all the bridal magazines had promised me. I was a bit of an emotional mess.

I looked in the mirror of my childhood bedroom and saw a fragmented version of myself: exhausted and worn down, twenty extra pounds of padding protecting my body from the insanity the year had brought, and a depleted, limp spirit that had drained away the sparkle in my eyes.

Most alarming of all, I had completely lost my love of music and singing. When Broadway went dark, a part of my heart went dark too. When I allowed music to flow through my body and throat, it was just a painful reminder of what I'd lost. It felt like water running into a pot with no drainage, pooling inside me and becoming stagnant with the rot of depression and anxiety.

My mom, an avid gardener and believer in nature as therapy, suggested I start walking in the forest each morning. I had recently read Dr. Li's book *Forest Bathing,* and decided it was time to put his practices to work and jump-start my emotional recovery from the pressures and transitions of the previous year.

It was in the daily repetition of those walks that I truly began to understand just how medicinal a forest can be. There is something about "forest silence," which isn't silent at all, that immediately relaxes your soul. In those walks, I allowed every emotion to rise and release: fear, anxiety, despair, helplessness—the works. I left all of them, and a lot of tears, in that forest.

Walking the same path became therapeutic in its own right. As I walked through the spring, summer, and fall of that year, I watched the forest grow and evolve on a daily basis. Every day there was a new animal, a new bloom, a new leaf to admire, a new season to experience.

Once an owl flew right overhead, perched in a tree, and initiated a staring contest with me for ten minutes. Another day I squatted in the middle of the walking path for ten minutes, observing a worm scoot its way across the ground. Have you ever really *watched* a worm? Watching its contortions is like getting a free ticket to Mother Nature's circus.

I became friends with the family of blue jays that greeted me several times a week with their song—or rather, shrieks. I'd often find myself stopped in my tracks, mesmerized by the colony of inchworms dangling from their translucent threads, dancing across the sky. In the forest, my troubles would drift away as I lost myself in the marvels of the natural world.

We had record storms that summer, and I watched trees fall and decompose and return to the soil. Staring at their damp, reddish, decomposing bodies, I'd contemplate their life cycles and smile at how generous it was of them to return to the soil as the food that their siblings and offspring would use to grow taller. After learning about the "wood wide web" of mycorrhizal fungi connecting the trees in the forest together through their root systems . . . I couldn't take a step without guessing how many thousands of superhighways were at work beneath my feet.

Slowly, as I put one step in front of the other, in the "quiet" of the forest I became reacquainted with that dormant corner of my heart, and felt spring gently nudging me back to life.

Day by day, the forest filled me back up. After a month or so of walking, I suddenly felt an internal spark of inspiration to sing. Initially, I'd control a quiet hum as I walked and observed the forest, mimicking birdsong or remembering favorite tunes. Eventually my hums turned into verses, which turned into full-voiced songs while the local birds joined in as backup singers. The walks soon became more than a way to work through anxiety and depression; they became a welcomed harbor of lightness I hadn't felt in months. The trees and birds not only held space for me to grieve and recoup after a crazy season of life, they became my audience and collaborators. I didn't go to the forest to find my voice again, but in the hours I spent there, my voice found me.

That's the magic of Forest Therapy: It clears the field, makes space for you to simply be. In that "being," the heaviness of life lifts and you find your pure self, your spirit, your inner—and sometimes literal—voice.

One Green Thing

As much as we need nature, nature also needs us right now. The potted plants we have in our home are only a small representation of the flora and fauna that make our planet inhabitable. As of 2021, the Convention on International Trade in Endangered Species of Wild Fauna and Flora (CITES) has over 38,700 species on its three appendices of threatened or endangered species. Of those, 32,800 of them are plant species.[17] That's 85 percent of the entire list. We must wake up and consider the importance of plants and the amazing things they do for us and our planet. On a large scale, they absorb carbon dioxide, release air for us to breathe, help purify water, and, of course, provide food for us to eat. On a smaller scale, they help us find stillness and solace in our busy workdays, reveal the fragility and beauty of life, and teach life lesson after life lesson, if we're receptive enough to notice them and learn.

As we learn how fragile our natural world is and begin to reap the rewards of a closer relationship with nature, the question becomes how we can protect the beauty around us. What is one shift you can make in your life to make the world a greener and cleaner place? Pick a time frame that feels reasonable for you—maybe once a month, or every three months—and focus on incorporating one environmentally friendly habit into your life.

It could be eliminating single-use plastics, evaluating the sustainability of your plant collection, or buying local produce. Whatever it is, focus on incorporating this earth-friendly practice into your day-to-day life. Once it has become part of your lifestyle, add another earth-friendly habit. Slowly but surely, that list of eco-friendly shifts you want to make will become integrated into your life, with no overwhelm necessary.

Get involved: Find a local group that's passionate about making a difference and join it. Whether it's volunteering at a community or school garden, participating in a neighborhood or beach cleanup, or helping with tree recovery or planting projects, you don't have to be alone in your efforts to help the planet. Volunteering with like-minded groups will help multiply your contribution and connect you with new, like-minded friends.

Engage Your Senses

Once you bring a plant home, you enter into a relationship with it. Observing your plants and learning about their needs through trial, error, and experience leads to an ongoing dialogue between you and your little green friends. You begin to listen, to tune your senses to understand what a plant needs. Plant care is not only a fun hobby, but an opportunity to help us develop and engage with our senses on a deeper level.

It's so easy to take our gifts of sight, smell, taste, hearing, and touch for granted as we automatically use them all day long. There are so many beautiful ways to enrich our relationship with the natural world and ourselves by heightening our senses. How can you describe the differences between the texture of a velvet philodendron (*Philodendron micans*) leaf and a heartleaf philodendron (*P. hederaceum*) leaf? How does a store-bought tomato taste compared with a home-grown one? What are the sounds that make up "forest silence"? **Let's grow some joy by deepening our relationship with plants beyond plain sight.**

See

Here are some fun practices to get you present, curious, and noticing the green world that surrounds us.

Look for love in your leaf shapes

Have you noticed that many tropical houseplant leaves are heart-shaped? Swiss cheese plant (*M. deliciosa*), heartleaf philodendron (*P. hederaceum*), and string of hearts (*Ceropegia woodii*) are three of my favorite heart-shaped plants in my collection.

OTHER FANTASTIC HEART-SHAPED HOUSEPLANTS

- heartleaf hoya (*Hoya kerrii*)
- *Philodendron gloriosum*
- cyclamen (*Cyclamen* spp.)
- flamingo flower (*Anthurium andraeanum*)
- heartleaf fern (*Hemionitis arifolia*)

Use your plants as a reminder to constantly cultivate feelings of love within yourself. **Keep heart-shaped plants scattered around your home, and every time you see them, send a little love to someone or something in your life, including you!**

Fill your collection with colorful foliage

The world of houseplants is so much wider than the common golden pothos (*Epipremnum aureum*) we remember from our grandparents' home. The plants that are available to us now come in all shapes, sizes, and colors. Consider bringing a plant with variegated or colorful foliage home to mix up the look of your collection. Besides, who can resist falling in love with the pink foliage on a *Philodendron* 'Pink Princess'? Just note that variegated or brightly colored plants have different care requirements, often requiring more light than their nonvariegated counterparts.

SOME COLORFUL PLANTS TO TRY AT HOME

- inch plant (*Tradescantia zebrina*)
- purple shamrock plant (*Oxalis triangularis* 'Charmed Wine')
- nerve plant (*Fittonia* spp.) comes in many different varieties with white, pink, or red veining
- polka dot plant (*Hypoestes phyllostachya*) is similar to the nerve plant but can grow taller, with larger leaves
- African violets (*Saintpaulia* spp.) come in a multitude of varieties with variegated or

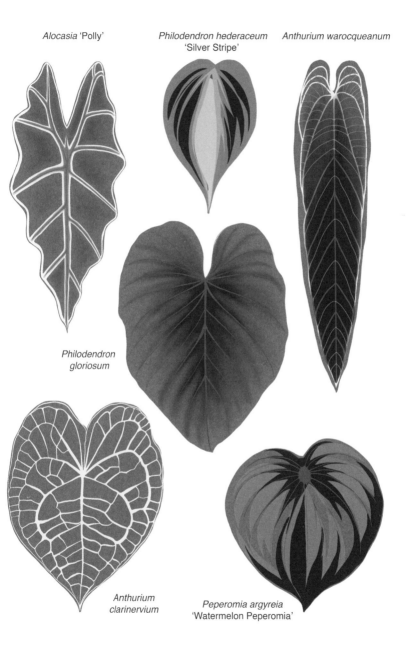

Alocasia 'Polly'

Philodendron hederaceum 'Silver Stripe'

Anthurium warocqueanum

Philodendron gloriosum

Anthurium clarinervium

Peperomia argyreia 'Watermelon Peperomia'

ruffled leaves and blooms in every color you can dream of

- the *Calathea* and *Maranta* genera both have beautifully patterned leaves, and many species have gorgeous purple undersides

- croton (*Codiaeum variegatum*) come in a variety of green, yellow, orange, and even pink varieties

- Succulents, if you dare, come in a mind-blowing variety of colors, even blue! Just make sure they are getting loads of sun and periods of drought if you try to keep them indoors.

Feature your plant of the month

Beyond heart shapes and colors, leaves come in the most amazing array of shapes and sizes. Once we start growing our plant collections, it's easy to see them as a whole and lose sight of the beauty in each and every plant we have. A great way to avoid this mistake is to pick a plant of the month—think employee of the month, but the planty version. Put your standout plant in a special spot where you'll see it (just make sure it still has the light it needs), dress it up with a particularly pretty cachepot, or make it the focal point of your décor for a bit. While your plant is "on stage," take the time to really notice it. Dig a little bit deeper and research its origins and care requirements, and the different propagation methods that work for it.

Appreciate the shape of its leaves, the colors on the leaves and stem, and new growth or fading leaves. Observe the growth patterns of the leaves: Do they alternate down the vine of a stem like a *Philodendron* 'Brasil'? Does the plant have just one leaf per stem like watermelon peperomia (*Peperomia argyreia*)? Maybe the leaves come in adorable triplets like on a *Peperomia* 'Hope' or purple shamrock plant (*Oxalis triangularis*). Celebrate your plant of the month; get curious and develop a deeper appreciation for its unique awesomeness.

Smell

Of all of our senses, smell is the most powerful and unique, because our nose is a straight shot to the part of our brain associated with long-term memories and emotions.[1] When we are in nature, we are benefiting not only from the view, but from the relaxing effects of the scent of trees and plants.

Fun fact: Most of the smells we associate with plants—fragrant roses, freshly cut grass, invigorating eucalyptus—are actually the plant's way of communicating with itself and its environment. Who knew!? Well, scientists did. Plants release VOCs (volatile organic compounds) through their epidermal tissue in order to ward off herbivores, attract a pollinator, or even communicate with other parts of itself or other plants around it.

Another fun, but sad, fact: That smell of fresh-cut grass we all know and love is actually the poor little blades alerting their other blade friends: "Intruder! We are being attacked! Beware!" Poor guys.[2]

Now that we've established that plant scents are more than just a fun thing to collect for your aromatherapy collection, let's talk about some fun plant smells and their effects on the human body—which will prove just how important scent can be in cultivating calm within your life.

Phytoncides are the VOCs emitted by trees (and other plants) to defend themselves against unwanted visitors like fungi, insects, and bacteria. Dr. Qing Li (yes, the aforementioned scientist I am obsessed with) discovered that research subjects who slept with hinoki stem cell oil diffused in the air slept longer and had decreased levels of stress hormones. Other studies have shown that the presence of phytoncides can lift your mood, lower your blood pressure, suppress your sympathetic nervous activity, and increase your parasympathetic nervous activity (the "rest and digest" vibes we are so hungry for).

Geosmin: You know that earthy, funky, invigorating smell outside after it rains? That intoxicating scent is petrichor, the effect of geosmin, a compound secreted by bacteria found in soil, which is released into the air after it rains. Humans are very sensitive to the presence of geosmin, likely because it is an indicator of the presence of water.

Go for a post-rain, restorative walk

There truly is nothing like the smell of the earth after a rainstorm. Thanks, geosmin! Next time it rains, take yourself for a (screen-free) walk around your block and take lots of luscious deep breaths. There is nothing like that sweet, post-rain silence and the rich fragrance of the earth.

Breathe deeply. Cultivate calm. Smile. Even if you step outside for only a quick moment, this practice can center you and wring your daily stress right out.

Essential oils

Although many of us would love to be frolicking in forests and gardens all day to reap the benefits of inhaling these fantastic aromas, unfortunately that's just not realistic. Most of us are stuck indoors at an office or desk. That doesn't mean we can't "hack" our way into enjoying the benefits of planty smells! Enter essential oils.

When it comes to choosing essential oils, my overall advice is "Choose what makes you feel good." The scent/brain connection is so personal, and this practice is all about finding more joy and less stress in your everyday life, so . . . pick scents that put a smile on your face or give you that relaxing rush that swooshes down your spine. Play around with several high-quality, pure essential oils and the diffusing method that works for your space, and mix and match until you find your perfect blend.

Mixing an oil blend to match your mood is a little routine to look forward to at the beginning of the day and sets the tone for how you show up. Keep several bottles of different scents next to your diffuser, and become a "mad scientist" for a moment to mix your scent of the day. For the last several months I've been on a major hinoki oil kick, but recently, I've been very drawn to lavender. There's no right answer, and nothing needs to stay the same. As with your plant collection, feel free to play with, change, and grow your selection of scents.

HOW TO DIFFUSE ESSENTIAL OILS

There are several ways to diffuse essential oils in your home: through a traditional diffuser (which requires a battery or electrical outlet), a reed diffuser (where oils are wicked up a diffuser reed or bamboo stick and passively dispersed in your home), or a candle. There are thousands of diffusers with all sorts of price points on the market, so choose what works for you and experiment!

It's up to you to choose which plant oils make your heart sing, but here are the go-to essential oils I like to diffuse in my home to help you get started:

- hinoki (*Chamaecyparis obstusa*), the oil Dr. Li used in the study mentioned earlier. It has an intoxicating lemony, woodsy scent that I enjoy using throughout the workday.

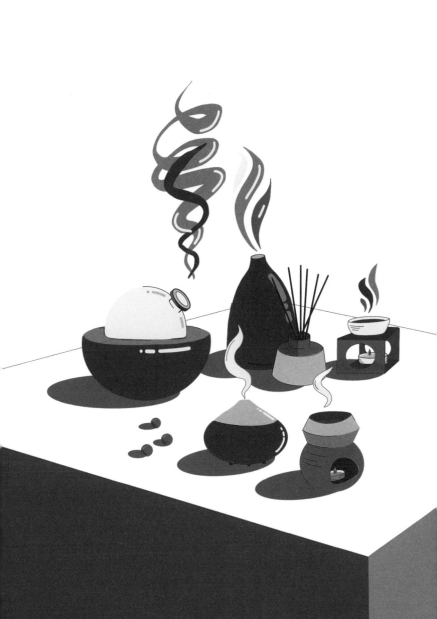

- lavender (*Lavandula* spp.), a tried-and-true soothing fragrance to calm any busy mind down and relieve stress and anxiety.[3, 4]

- rosemary (*Salvia rosmarinus*), one of my favorites, has the most refreshing, stimulating scent.

- eucalyptus (*Eucalyptus globulus*) immediately gives a spa-like feeling to any area of your home.

- cedarwood (*Cedrus atlantica*) is like a woodsy, warm hug.

- thieves oil, a warm, spicy blend of clove, lemon, cinnamon, rosemary, and eucalyptus. Many people use thieves in their homemade cleaning solutions.

Note, essential oils don't work for everyone, as we are all unique snowflakes. Some people have intense smell aversions, and oil perfume is too much for them. More important, in some cases essential oils can cause allergic contact dermatitis when applied to the skin. Consult a doctor if you feel you are having an allergic reaction.

Add fragrant plants to your indoor plant collection

Take plant parenthood to the next level by picking plants based on scent in addition to appearance and care requirements. Keeping potted lavender, herbs, or plants such as orchids and hoya that have famously fragrant blooms will grow you many joyful moments. Sneak scent breaks with your plants throughout the day. Break off a leaf or bloom and inhale for a few seconds to be transported wherever that scent memory takes you. I love keeping basil inside, because it reminds me of my mom. Here are some other lovely scented plants to play around with. Remember, scent is personal, so choose what makes you happy, and check the care guides for your preferred plants before bringing them home.

FABULOUSLY SCENTED PLANTS

- lavender (*Lavandula* spp.)
- rosemary (*Salvia rosmarinus*)
- basil (*Ocimum basilicum*)
- mint (*Mentha* spp.), my favorite to wake up with in the morning
- *Hoya lacunosa*, blooms smell like cinnamon
- *Hoya* sp. aff. *burtoniae*, blooms are said to smell like buttered popcorn
- *Hoya carnosa*, blooms smell like chocolate
- *Maxillaria tenuifolia*, nicknamed "The Coconut Orchid" for its piña colada scented blooms that would make anyone smile
- Rose-scented geranium (*Pelargonium graveolens*), the plants we know and love as

scented geraniums, actually aren't geraniums but rather *Pelargonium* spp. They come in all sorts of scent varieties and many of the leaves can be used in cooking or added to any bath to turn it from a normal bath to full-out spa; just add sliced cucumbers to your eyes and you're basically treating yourself to a fancy spa day for free!

- Hyacinth (*Hyacinthus orientalis*): Nothing says spring like the sweet scent of hyacinth.

Long commutes? Grow joy on your dashboard

My mom, an avid gardener and lavender grower, snips fresh bundles of lavender that she then places on her car dashboard. As the sun heats the lavender, it spreads the relaxing scent throughout her car and makes for the most delightful drive, no matter how long the journey might be.

Sounds of the Forest

Silence is a sacred and scarce commodity in the United States. There are very few places that aren't affected by noise pollution. When I lived in New York City, I was lucky to be a sound enough sleeper that the speeding cars on the nearby highway and random 4 A.M. construction crews and garbage trucks never woke me. My sweet partner was not so lucky, and needed to sleep with foam earbuds every night. When we moved to five acres in the middle of the woods, the silence was deafening. I only truly understood the concept of sound pollution, and how accustomed I had grown to NYC's "white noise," after I experienced its absence. My body and nervous system were so unused to being in the quiet, it actually triggered anxiety.

In those first few weeks in our new home, we'd look at each other and marvel at how quiet it was outside. I couldn't stop listening to the crescendo of wind rustling in the trees and the beautiful soprano trills of the local bird chatter. As I began to unwind from my unwittingly noisy lifestyle, I slowly felt my entire being relax and embrace a level of calm I had thought was only reserved for vacations. It felt like my entire body unclenched a little bit, even though I'd never realized it was tense to begin with. We've grown accustomed to the ambient noise of cars, factories, and construction, but our nervous systems simply have not.[5]

No one understands this better than Gordon Hempton, an acoustic ecologist known as "The Sound Tracker®." He travels the world capturing disappearing natural soundscapes and is known for his fight to preserve the natural soundscape of "one square inch" of Hoh Rain Forest in Olympic National Park, which Hempton has described as the quietest place in the country. Hempton predicts that natural silence could become extinct in the next ten years unless action is taken to preserve it.[6] If you visit onesquareinch.org you can enjoy a fifteen-minute recording of the natural soundscape. When

> **IT IS OUR BIRTHRIGHT TO LISTEN, QUIETLY AND UNDISTURBED, TO THE NATURAL ENVIRONMENT AND TAKE WHATEVER MEANINGS WE MAY FROM IT.**

—GORDON HEMPTON

you hit "play" and the sound of trickling water and crickets tickles your ears, get ready to feel a relaxing whoosh run down your spine like water running over a river stone.

If you are chasing some silence of your own, you can visit the exact square inch at Olympic National Park. It's marked by a red stone on top of a moss-covered log at N 48.12885°, W 123.68234°, 303 feet above sea level.

Since we can't put traffic, running refrigerators, washer/ dryers, or flight paths on mute, drowning them out with recordings of natural sounds is our next best option, as well as a fun way to bring the outside in.[7] You can find recordings of natural soundscapes easily on Spotify, YouTube, or Gordon's website. I found an eight-hour YouTube video of nature sounds that I play throughout my workday. Once the recording is over, I know the eight-hour workday is up and it's time to disconnect from my computer.

The sounds of the rain forest have underscored my entire writing process for this book, and personally, I find that I'm always more focused and productive when listening to sounds of the forest and birdsong, compared with sitting in office silence.

Ideas for incorporating natural soundscapes into your home

- If you live in a natural area, open your windows to allow the songs of your local wildlife in.

- Program your alarm to wake you with birdsong instead of an intrusive beep. Birdsong has been proven to reduce levels of cortisol in the body[8] and is just so darn delightful.
- Underscore your workday with your favorite sounds of nature.
- Add a small water feature at your desk to enjoy the sound of trickling water.
- Put on nature-inspired music playlists while you cook dinner.
- Sleep with a white-noise machine that plays rain forest or ocean sounds.

When we consider how disconnected we are from the natural world, we need to remember we are as aurally disconnected as we are visually. So find some "quiet" and listen; open your world up to the delightful "forest silence" and the physical and emotional response that will unfold.

Feel Your Plants, Feel Your Feels

In the "See" section, we talked about how noticing the shapes and growing patterns of our plants can be an easy way to better understand and appreciate them. Touch is another incredibly powerful sense we can engage with.

Look around your plant collection and feel your plants. The raised almost leathery feel of a *Monstera* sp. Peru[9] leaf is so different from the wispy, delicate lace-like leaves of a maidenhair fern (*Adiantum raddianum*), which contrasts to the velvety texture of the velvet leaf philodendron (*P. micans*) leaf. Some plants have developed thorns or spines to ward off predators. My lime tree wards me off every time I bump into him, by piercing my skin with his angry spines—a small price to pay for the joy of harvesting fresh limes for mojitos from our living room.

Feel your leaves. The tactile experience will bring you into the present and with luck instill a little awe as you marvel at Mother Nature's design sense.

Get your hands dirty

Plant people wear dirt under their fingernails as a badge of honor. There is no better, more visceral way to connect with nature than by good old-fashioned playing in the dirt.

Use your finger to monitor the water levels in your houseplants. Instead of jamming your hand in the potting mix and immediately deciding to water or not to water, turn this into a mindful moment. Notice the change in temperature as your finger digs beneath the soil. Damp soil tends to feel cooler to the touch than dry. Notice how compact the soil is and how much force it takes to break it up. When you pull your finger out of the soil, rub the earth between your fingers and feel the sensation of the exfoliation of tiny grains.

Set your pot-bound plants free

Repotting plants is one of the most fun, tactile ways we can get down and dirty with our plant collections. That being said, only repot plants if they *need* to be repotted. It's time to repot your plant if it needs fresh potting mix, a smaller container to combat overwatering and root decay, or, conversely, has become "pot-bound," meaning that the root mass has become too large for the pot. Some species may need repotting annually, while others are content in the same pot for longer. You'll notice that a plant is pot-bound if the roots are growing out of the hole in the bottom of the pot, if you take the plant out of its pot and see the roots growing in concentric circles over each other in the shape of the bottom of the pot, or if the plant continually dries out, even with frequent watering. This is not good for the plant, as the roots need to rest in soil to be able to uptake water and nutrients.

When your plant becomes pot-bound, you need to set those roots free by potting the plant up in a larger pot. Best practice is to choose a pot that's two inches larger than the current one. If you are a newbie, be careful here: Lots of new plant parents pot their plants in containers way too large for the existing root system, which can lead to root rot and fungal issues. So never bump a tropical houseplant up from a 4-inch pot to a 10-inch pot. A 6-incher should be a fantastic home upgrade for your growing green friend.

Before you put your plant in its new pot, it's important to free the roots by getting your hands in that root mass and loosening the tight pattern the roots are currently growing in. If the roots break, fear not! This will trigger them to grow more. If you don't shimmy those roots out of the pattern they're growing in, they might continue to grow in that shape, even in their new, roomier home.

There are always exceptions to these rules: Some species of plants perform better when somewhat pot-bound. These are species that don't tolerate a lot of excess moisture at the root zone in a pot, or that need to dry faster between waterings. Epiphytic species such as orchids or bromeliads that are potted may also be fine when they appear pot-bound, as they wouldn't normally have their root system totally surrounded by soil or other growing media.

Dig Deep

Do you feel pot-bound in any area of your life? Are any habits or growth patterns inhibiting your ability to flourish and thrive? As you repot your plants, consider how you might go about setting yourself free as well. Remember that breaking old patterns brings new growth!

Get your ground on

Grounding is a therapeutic practice that is said to reconnect our body's electrical energy with the natural electric current of the earth. The surface of the earth is a vast supply of electrons that we can connect to through the soles of our feet, but shoes have really cramped this energy transfer's style. Now that walking barefoot isn't common practice, we are disconnected from this delightful source of energy and connection with the natural world.

TRY GROUNDING FOR YOURSELF

On your lawn or in a nearby park, spend five minutes with your feet on the ground and delight in the tickle of the grass as it slides between your toes. Visualize yourself as a tree growing roots deep into the earth, stand tall, and face the sun. Take deep breaths and allow yourself to have an exquisite moment of connection with the earth and yourself.

Taste: Grow Your Own Food . . . Then Sample It

So many of us are disconnected from the food we eat. I'm sure you know at least one person who couldn't tell you how cashews grow or what an eggplant flower looks like or that herbs don't come from small plastic boxes in the refrigerated section of the grocery store. Growing your own food, even if it's just a small planter of herbs, is the most empowering feeling. It also happens to empower your bank account with all the money you save on those pricey containers of wilted basil at the grocery store. Some of my most cherished family memories are picking tomatoes off my mom's tomato plants with my sister, and watching my mom flail a zucchini the size of a turkey leg in the air, shouting in delight at the enormous harvest. She'd then take those zucchini flowers, coat them in flour, and fry them in olive oil, like my Italian cousins do, to feel more connected to them, even if we are oceans away.

Herbs were our gateway drug into plant parenthood. My journey to "Happy Plant Lady" started with a small planter of herbs on our balcony. That summer, Billy took our homegrown basil and made pints of pesto so delicious I ate it with a spoon. Snipping chives to scramble into my eggs became a welcome addition to my morning practice. Our meals were elevated by our herbal garnishes, and we felt new ownership over the meals we were making because we were responsible for growing some of the food we were enjoying.

For people who love slower-growing, tropical house-plants, growing harvestable plants is also a fun way to ex-perience a faster life cycle. In many cases you can see a plant go from seed to harvest in a few short months, while we might wait a year for a monstera leaf to pop up and unfurl.

Figure out what plants you want to eat, and grow some joy for your taste buds as well as your soul.

Here are some ways you can grow your own food:

Balcony or windowsill herb garden

- Choose the sunniest spot on your balcony or in your yard or the sunniest southern-facing windowsill you've got. Herbs need six to eight hours of direct sunlight. If you don't have direct light in your home, you can supplement it with a grow light. See the section on grow lights in the back of the book.

- Select several healthy, pest-free seedlings of your favorite herbs and pot them in terra-cotta pots with drainage holes or alongside each other in a longer planter. Always keep mint in a pot of its own, because it's overly friendly.

- Use a potting mix, not your garden soil. You want a mix that drains quickly and doesn't give your herbs "wet feet." This is why it's also important to use pots with holes at the bottom, to allow excess water to escape.

- Once your herbs are established and have grown large enough, it's harvest time! I recommend avoiding harvesting more than a third of the plant at a time. If you notice your herbs flowering, pinch the flowers off so the plant focuses on growing more tasty leaves.

- If plants get leggy (elongated and limp) it means they aren't getting enough light. Prune them back by up to 50 percent to trigger new lateral growth, and move to a location with more sun or a grow light.

Hydroponic garden

If you aren't a fan of soil, but want to get your grow on, hydroponic gardening is a great option. Hydroponic gardening is the soil-less cultivation of plants using only water with a nutrient solution, or an inorganic substrate for support, and a pump. You grow your plants in pods made up of inorganic material like coco coir, vermiculite, or perlite. The plant gets its food by absorbing the nutrient-rich water solution.

Because you control the nutrients and lighting when growing hydroponically indoors, you have a lot of control over what you grow. If the nutrients and lighting are right, you can grow delicious lettuce, herbs, strawberries, or even tomatoes indoors, regardless of the season. Hydroponic gardening on a large scale isn't easy and requires lots of mixing of nutrient solutions and tinkering with grow lights. If you're curious, I suggest starting off with one of the many "plug and play" hydroponic setups on the market; they can be small enough to fit on a kitchen counter or as large as a bookshelf.

It's mid-January as I write this book, with two feet of snow outside, and I currently have a five-foot-tall hydroponic system with grow lights that is growing basil, parsley, oregano, thyme, sage, cilantro, viola flowers, spinach, kale, broccoli, bok choy, tatsoi, sugar snap peas, and two microdwarf tomato plants. The system takes up less than two square feet of floor space. I call it my "Spaceship Smoothie Tower," and it's pretty awesome. In the middle of winter, surrounded by snow and low light, I get to watch my snap peas go from vine, to flower, to tiny pea, to tasty treat. I harvest greens for my daily smoothie fresh from my living room every morning. It doesn't get more locally grown than that!

Join a community garden

If you're in a city, you can look up your community garden and reserve a plot for yourself to not only grow some delicious food, but to grow a deeper connection with your neighbors. I never belonged to a community garden when I lived in NYC . . . but I stalked one daily on my morning walks. This secret garden was tucked away on the Long Island City waterfront, and beyond a gate were eight raised beds filled with gorgeous flowers, herbs, tomatoes, and vegetables. I'd visit the garden every day and stroll through the beds to see what was growing. I had many delightful conversations with the garden owners about what they enjoyed growing, and asked them for tips for my more modest balcony garden back home.

How to find your local community garden, you ask? Google is your best friend here. Search your zip code and "community garden" and get clicking.

Taste-test your homegrown vs. store-bought produce

Although most gardeners will wax poetic about the unbelievable difference in taste between a homegrown and a store-bought tomato—a difference that is totally real, by the way—you can try this practice with almost any edible plant you want to grow. Packaged, store-bought basil begins to lose its flavor and alluring scent immediately after it's been cut from its mother plant. The Boston Bibb lettuce I grow in my hydroponic tower is sweeter, crunchier, and has a more complex flavor profile than any head of lettuce I've ever bought at the store. When I tasted the homegrown version, it felt like I was tasting lettuce for the first time!

Compare your homegrown harvest with options purchased from the grocery store, or even do a blind taste test to see if you can tell the difference! Think of your homegrown cucumber or rosemary as a fine wine or complex chocolate, and pay attention as you eat it. What flavors do you experience? Does it differ in texture from its store-bought counterpart? How does the flavor change from beginning to end—what do you taste first, and what lingers?

Grow Your Own Way: A Lesson from My Herb Garden

A modest herb garden can be a big teacher. Not only will it inspire you to learn different recipes to impress your partners and friends at the dinner table, but if you observe the herbs over a season of growth, you can learn a thing or two about your *own* growth. My favorite herbs to grow are: basil, sage, chives, oregano, thyme, and mint. I grow them alongside each other in long rectangular planters, with the exception of mint, which gets its own container because of its overly enthusiastic personality. Throughout the season I observe all the plants grow larger, but although they thrive together, if you look closely enough you will notice that they grow very differently.

There's Basil, my slow, steady, and sensitive friend. Basil starts out as this tiny little guy, growing bit by bit, millimeter by millimeter, until he is towering over the rest of his companions. He is the star of the herb garden; who doesn't love homemade pesto or a chiffonade of basil on top of a slice of pizza?! And don't even get me started on his scent—it's intoxicating. If there was a perfume made out of basil, I'd wear it.

Although Basil is a star, he's definitely a gentle giant—though he can be a bit of a diva when it comes to watering and temperature. If it's too hot or if it's been too long since his last drink, he'll throw a little fit and wilt dramatically,

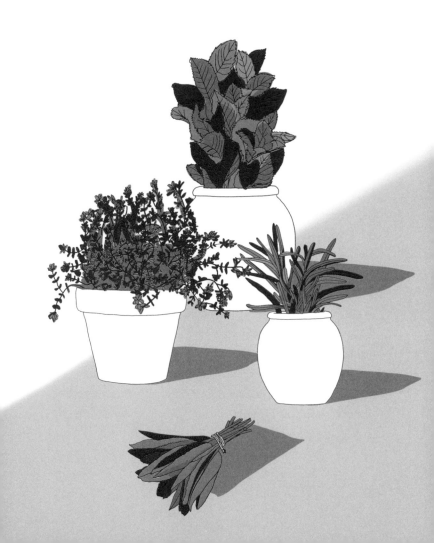

looking for attention. But, with some attention, he faithfully perks right back up and continues to grow a bountiful supply of the delicious leaves I will never get enough of.

Next to him is sturdy Sage. She also grows centimeter by centimeter, but in a steady way that makes her incredibly hardy. There is not a trace of diva in her; she's a salt-of-the-earth type of lady. She will be the first to wake up and show her leaves in the spring, and she'll continue to blow me away by surviving cold snaps in the fall, even hanging on through a bit of snow before she goes back to sleep for the winter. She's quieter; she knows her time to shine is later in the season when we prepare for more savory, heartier meals, and she's okay with that. Steady Sage is a master class in resilience and patience.

Thyme believes in strength in numbers, with her tiny leaves tumbling over the planter—delicate, fragrant, and incredibly versatile. Chives make no apologies for their towering, no-frills appearance and their straight-to-the-point flavor that can knock your socks off.

And then there's good old, friendly, slightly spastic Mint. Mint is an unpredictable maverick who would take over the whole balcony garden if I let him. I keep Mint in a separate container, knowing his gregarious tendencies, but he loves company so much that one summer, against all odds and means of separation, Mint actually found a way to jump from his lonely circular container into the rectangular one with all of his friends. Mint is wild and unpredictable, and you need to make sure you rein him in occasionally; but he's a friend you can count on to show up at your party no matter what.

Within a singular season, these deliciously fragrant herbs all grow successfully but have different growth habits, shine uniquely, and *not one of them gives a shit about what the other plants are doing.* How badass is that?

I think about these herbs and their different growing styles when I catch myself getting caught in the comparison game with others around me. It's so easy to compare and contrast yourself with others and feel bad about your lack of accomplishments. I've lost hours of my life looking at other people's curated photos, their perceived accomplishments and humble brags that make me fear that I'm too far behind and will never catch up. It's so easy to feel inadequate when you let social media, the leaders of the PTA, or members of your family dictate how you live your life and what your definition of success is. Think about the time we've lost obsessing over person X's perceived wins, when we could have taken that time to actually fuel it into our own creativity and success! *face-palm*

There is room at the table for everyone; each individual is on his or her own journey of growth and development, like my herbs. You will pull ahead, you will fall behind, you will get pruned, you will face adversity, you will have wins to brag about, and you'll also have losses.

The secret is that you're exactly where you need to be, in your container of planted humanity, whether you realize it or not. So instead of stressing about who is growing the tallest, smelling the most fragrant, or climbing into the most pots, how about celebrating exactly where you are, rooted in this moment? Be kind to yourself like you're kind to your plants. Trust that you're on track to grow and bloom and (figuratively) die back when the timing is right. Yes, it takes patience and trust; but the wait is half the fun, isn't it?

Dig Deep

What herb are you?

Pick your favorite herb and imagine yourself as that herb growing like the ones in the story above. So who are you? Slow and steady Basil? Wild and unpredictable Mint? Resilient Sage? How can you identify and celebrate your own growth patterns? Pick one and run with it. Breathe into how silly you feel and then release it.

Visualize your roots: Think about where you've been and how far you've come.

Breathe into the appreciation of the people in your life who lift you up and support you like the soil that surrounds your roots.

Imagine yourself, leaves pointed toward the sun, growing and expanding. Taking up space. You are exactly where you need to be.

Here are some journaling prompts for you to explore:

- What is one area of my life I've grown in this year/six months/week?
- Who am I comparing myself with or envious of? How can I reframe their success and make it a source of inspiration instead of jealousy? How can I celebrate their growth?
- Who am I "planted" with, and how do they make me feel?
- What do I want to grow into?

Take a few deep breaths, look inward, and celebrate yourself, you little herb you!

THE SECRET
IS THAT YOU'RE
EXACTLY
WHERE YOU
NEED TO BE.

Plant Seeds
of Delight

When I was a kid my best friend Jackie and I would play outside in her backyard every day. Jackie and I had limitless imaginations; we'd go on adventures far beyond the scope of her parents' address. One day we'd be explorers traversing the stone wall along her property line, collecting vacated cicada shells as "treasure." The next day we'd be Secret Service agents collecting information on Mark, the older boy next door, planning a water balloon war to wage on him and save the planet. We had little regard for what the cool kids were into back then.

Frankly, we were pretty weird. Jackie, nicknamed "Wacky Jackie," was a natural athlete, tomboy, and wild spirit who had a healthy obsession with books filled with ghost stories that had the other girls in our class spooked. I, the ahead-of-her-time fashionista, wore blue leopard-print bell-bottoms and corralled my unruly bangs into a small unicorn horn–like ponytail at the front of my head to keep them out of my face. In hindsight, it was practical, but never became a trend the popular girls copied.

Regardless of what the other kids thought of us, Jackie

and I thought we were awesome. We followed our instincts, enjoyed our imaginations, indulged our curiosity, and really let our inner freak flags fly together.

The best adventures were when we would make feasts for imaginary guests out of the materials we found in her backyard: salads of grass and holly berries, platters of wild and pungent onion grass, and pies made out of mud and whatever other things were "in season." We had no fear when it came to engaging our five senses in our playtime, and no concern for the mud and grass stains our poor mothers had to deal with at the end of the day. Sorry about that, Mom.

Plants are the new mud pies: an opportunity to engage our senses, enjoy the wonderful tactile experience of life, reconnect to our imaginations, and grow our own inner worlds and fill them up with joyful, playful moments.

Remember when in the beginning of this book I said to keep an open mind? That was for this section. You were warned! In this section, we shift from plant-*based* practices to plant-*inspired* practices. I'm going to encourage you to play and cultivate curiosity like your five-year-old self used to do in the playground. For some reason, as adults, we've lost touch with the imaginations we had as kids. Society has conditioned us to shed them like old, yellow leaves. It's a

PLANTS ARE THE NEW MUD PIES

real bummer, because having an imagination and "playing" is the best! Why that sense of expansion and amusement is reserved for children is beyond me. I think we should get over it and just keep playing until we die, not just until we go to college. Being "grown up" is overrated.

The practices in this next section might be a little "out there" or "woo-woo" or just plain unicorn-ponytail weird. But! They're also fun, uplifting, and an invitation to reconnect with your inner playful child. Do you want to be "cool" or do you want to be happy?

"~~Crazy~~ Happy Plant Lady"

As houseplants become more and more popular, many have said that the "Crazy Plant Lady" is the new "Crazy Cat Lady." We've all seen the memes and cartoons of the "Crazy Plant Lady": a woman surrounded by plants—with that *look in her eye*—as she proclaims that she can't socialize with other humans on a Saturday night because she has to stay home and water her plants instead. Bullshit. Listen . . . I'm what society would consider a "Crazy Plant Lady." I've got a whole lot of plants, and a whole lot of seemingly crazy love for them—but finding joy in cultivating life does not make you crazy. It makes you human. It also makes you happy.

I'm calling bullshit on this "Crazy Plant Lady" trend. We need a rebrand. "Crazy" isn't a word we should throw around so casually. I'm skipping "crazy" and sticking with

"~~Crazy~~ *Happy* Plant Lady." Houseplants, flowers, gardens, herbs, trees, and all the other green things in life make people happy. Plain and simple. So enough with the "crazy" and more of the "happy"!

Embrace your plant-loving, mud-pie-making self and let's unapologetically grow some joy!

Talk to Your Plants

Okay, before you immediately start rolling your eyes at me with this practice . . . give it a chance. The first time I talked about my experience with "planty affirmations" with my community of plant friends on Instagram, I was *sure* I was going to get laughed off the internet and have my "Plant Lady" title revoked. But I was keeping a secret I needed to share: I had these odd urges to speak and sing to my plants. And when I did, it felt good. Like audibly, literally, laugh-out-loud good. I'd sit on my balcony and tell my plants how lovely they looked, how proud I was of their growth, and sometimes I'd even rewrite songs to accommodate different herbs' names. Those moments made me smile, giggle, and be fully present.

And here's the thing: Whenever I post about this practice on social media, I am always *shocked* at how many people fess up to doing the same thing. So although this might be the silliest practice in the book, I hope it's the one that brings the biggest smile to your face!

Planty Affirmations, Two Ways

Affirmations are talked about by many of the best wellness gurus in the biz. They are said to lift your spirits, increase your confidence, help you overcome limiting beliefs, and just generally make you feel good. Marie Forleo tells a wonderful story about her book *Everything is Figureoutable*. She wrote "I am a NY Times Best Selling Author" fifteen times a day the entire time she was writing the book. It became a top seller! This shit works.

Sometimes it's uncomfortable to look in a mirror and say kind things to ourselves. But it's definitely easy to say something nice to your plant. Saying kind things to your plants will make you feel good, will probably make you giggle (because you're straight-up talking to a PLANT—how can that not bring a smile to your face!), and will instigate some warm and fuzzy bonding feelings between you and your collection. Connect to your inner nurturer and delight in what unfolds.

Our plant collections can be a mirror, a reflection of where we are in life. I've often found when my plants are struggling, I am too. There are so many garden/life parallels we can see and use every day to help *ourselves* grow, in addition to our plant collections. My hope is that after you affirm your plants, it will get easier and easier to say those affirmations to yourself. Next time you're brushing your teeth, prepping for the day, or struggling with overwhelm or anxiety about the future, try one of these on yourself and enjoy the warm fuzzies that will come along with it.

Affirmations to Try on Your Plants

- You grow, girl!
- Keep growing, plant friend!
- I'm proud of you, plant pal!
- I honor your dormancy and trust you will awaken at your perfect time.
- Unfurl your beautiful leaves and expand to your greatest potential.
- Everyone is growing at their own rate, in their right time; you're the exact right size and shape for this moment. Keep going. Keep growing.
- Stand tall and let yourself bloom, little plant!
- In this stillness, you grow.
- You are deserving of love, nutrients, and kindness.
- There is space in stillness.
- It's okay to lose leaves—let go of what doesn't serve you.

Planty Affirmations for You

- I'm growing and I'm doing great.
- I'm so proud of myself.
- Dormancy is okay. My next season will be full of growth and flowers.
- I'm an unfurling leaf, expanding into my greatest potential.
- I'm growing at my own rate, like everyone else is. I'm exactly where I need to be.
- Bloom unapologetically, baby!
- In this stillness, I'm still growing.
- I deserve love, nourishment, and kindness.
- There is space in stillness.
- It's okay to let things go. I'm letting go of what doesn't serve me anymore.
- Exciting seeds are germinating within me.

See them to believe them

Write these affirmations on notecards or Post-its and place them around your plants or on your bathroom mirror or refrigerator. Read them to yourself every time you pass them. The cumulative effect of this practice is pretty mind-blowing—say them daily, plant seeds of confidence within yourself, and marvel as they grow.

Name Your Plants

Naming your plants feels like the epitome of every Plant Lady parody you've ever seen . . . but it is so freaking fun. It makes you feel silly . . . but silly feels good. Try it. Worst comes to worst, the names don't stick. You don't have to name every plant in your collection; you can start with just one. But by naming your plants and personifying them a bit, you might just tap into a new level of nurturing and bonding that you wouldn't have experienced otherwise. I dare you not to smile while you call your plant by their name and give them a compliment.

I have named only some of my ninety-plus plants:

Limey the Bearss lime tree (*Citrus* x *latifolia* 'Bearss Seedless')

Lemony Snickett, my Meyer lemon tree (*Citrus* x *meyeri*)

Figaro the fiddle leaf fig (*Ficus lyrata*)

Gaga the MONSTERa (*M. deliciosa*)

I don't feel moved to name all of my plants, but a few extra-special plants needed names when they joined the collection. Limey was the first plant that Billy and I really took ownership of *together*. We harvested a lime and it became a delicious mojito. Once I was able to show how practical our plant collection could be, it was easier for Billy to appreciate my new and unexpected hobby. Figaro was the first plant that Billy brought home after a six-month "plant pause" that you'll learn about later in the book. Gaga is my little monster of a grower and named after our queen, Lady Gaga. Naming doesn't need to be rocket science; it's just plain fun.

Name your plants, grow some joy, and enjoy the smiles that spread across your face because of it.

The Ultimate Combo

Take one plant and give it your own name. Speak your planty affirmations to it. Every time you nurture your namesake plant and speak kindly to it, you'll be speaking kindly to your (secret) self. Suggestion: Choose a plant you already know how to take care of. The last thing you want is for your namesake plant not to love your home environment!

Learn the Latin

There are so many overlapping common names of plants, it's easy to get confused about what you are actually growing in your collection. A "friendship plant" could be *Pilea peperomioides* or *Pilea involucrata*. The term "ivy" is used in the common names of many tropical houseplants and outdoor vines of lots of different species. If you want to get serious about plant care, learning the Latin names of your plants is the best way to set yourself up for success. Don't get hung up on the pronunciation; no one pronounces plant Latin correctly.

Intimidated by those long, foreign names? An easy way to let them sink into your skull is to make little labels of the species' names for each of your plants and to stick them on the pots of your plants, so that every time you water them you can repeat the name to yourself, until finally you won't be able to *not* refer to your plants by their correct taxonomy! Plus, rattling off plant Latin is an easy way to look super fancy when you drag your friends plant-shopping.

Next-Level Joy Growing: Singing to Your Plants

This may be the most out-there thing I suggest: Sing to your plants. I know it sounds a little wackadoo, but it is SO FUN. Let their botanical beauty fill you with inspiration to search for botanically inspired music to sing around them. This is next-level "Happy Plant Lady" behavior, but man it feels good, and has me giggling by the end of every session.

Make your own song

Take your favorite song and rewrite it to include your plant. My favorite rewrite was for my oregano plant several summers ago. I took the chorus of Kesha's song "Blow" and changed the lyrics from "This place's about to blow, ooooohhohohoh" to "You grow, Orega-noooo-ohohohohoh." Did I look like a true weirdo to any neighbors or passersby on the street? Yep. Did I giggle to myself all day because of that moment and grow a little more joy in my life? Hell yes.

Here are some botanically inspired tunes to get you in the mood if you don't fancy yourself a song writer:

- "Edelweiss," from *The Sound of Music*
- "Back to the Garden," *Delta Rae*
- "The Secret Life of Plants," Stevie Wonder (This entire album is amazing.)
- "Grow As We Go," Ben Platt
- "(It's Not Easy) Bein' Green," Kermit the Frog (written by Joe Raposo)
- "Grow," Andy Grammer

Find Your Muse

You don't have to literally sing to your plants to enjoy this practice. Find the music—or painting or poem—within you, and let your plants inspire you creatively and artistically in a new way. If you have a spark of an idea, follow it.

Here are some ideas to get your creative juices flowing:

- What creative skills do you have that you've been wanting to explore more?

- If you can draw or paint, try sketching your favorite plant or botanical scene.

- Are you musical? Write a melody inspired by the sound of water coming through your watering can. What would it sound like if you could hear a leaf unfurl or a flower blossom?

- Are you a writer? Write botanically inspired poems, haikus, or short stories. Try capturing a scene inspired by nature—perhaps the way the light broke through the trees on your walk or the way leaves flutter in the wind.

- Take yourself on a planty artist date. The book *The Artist's Way* by Julia Cameron has sold millions of copies and helped countless people around the world reconnect with their inner artist. In the book, Julia suggests you take yourself on "artist dates," dedicated blocks of time to nurture your inner artist. We can easily take a note from Julia and find botanically inspired self-care dates for ourselves to reconnect with nature and our curiosity by visiting botanical gardens, finding art exhibitions centered on nature, trying out an art class on botanical illustration, or taking yourself on a Forest Bathing excursion.

Don't let your conditioned "adult" judge your creativity. Allow your inner child out to experiment and play.

Feel Spring in Your Body

Has your spirit ever felt dormant? Have you ever experienced seasons where you just can't get excited, or can't get your energy moving? Try embodying spring.

This practice is inspired by the energizing changing of the seasons from winter to spring. In New York, when March rolls around, there is a palpable shift in energy as the first warm spring days approach. You can feel the barren trees waking up and almost hear buds forming. Glimmers of green are everywhere after a dark gray, dormant winter. A sense of promise hangs in the air, heavy with excitement for the warmth, growth, and Summer Fridays to come.

This practice is simple. Turn on your favorite dance music and visualize a spring awakening in your body. Let yourself move to the rhythm. Take whatever visuals of spring are the most resonant for you and feel them within your body. It could be a seed germinating and poking forth its first true leaves, a tender bud forming, a daffodil blooming. Use whatever imagery inspires you and let the moves and energy flow.

PS: Adding this practice to your morning routine is a delightful way to wake up your body and mind to start your day.

Celebrate Your Plant/Life Parallels

When I started caring for plants, I began to see aspects of my own life reflected in my plant collection. There are lots of lessons to be learned from the parallels between our plants' lives and our own. My sign-off for my podcast is "Keep Blooming and Keep Growing." Yes, this is cheesy, but it's also a very powerful mantra. Plants are our green teachers, showing us simple, natural truths we often lose sight of. In this chapter you'll find a few powerful lessons and some dig-deeper prompts for you to use. I share my lessons in hopes that you find parallels in your own life that will help you on your journey.

Make a Pruning List

The concept of pruning seems counterintuitive: Cut something back and make it smaller in order to help it grow into a lusher, fuller plant than it would have been without a little growth-inspiring haircut. Cut one flower now, get two flowers later. The science behind pruning is even cooler.

To understand pruning you need to know about a hormone called auxin and a part of the plant called the apical meristem. Auxin is one of the primary hormones responsible for a lot of important stuff that goes on in a plant, such as shoot, root, and fruit growth. A plant has an apical meristem in the terminal, or tippity-top, bud. And the buds are where the growth happens.

The terminal bud, which houses the apical meristem, is the boss. It regulates the auxin distribution throughout the plant, thus regulating plant growth and development in conjunction with other phytohormones. When you remove a terminal bud, you are essentially removing the regulator of the auxin, triggering all of those lateral buds to grow.

There have been difficult seasons of my life when not a day went by that I didn't think of pruning. When I worried about whatever was being "pruned away"—a job, my wedding date, a home—I'd take three deep breaths and remind myself of the robust growth, better flowers, and beautiful new foliage that comes after a pruning. I was able to reframe and to focus on the exciting growth that would come in the future.

WHEN YOU'RE STRUGGLING WITH LOSS OR FEAR, TRY THIS MANTRA:

"After pruning, comes new growth"

"After pruning, comes new growth"

"After pruning, comes new growth"

Dig Deep

What have you pruned back in your life that allowed you to reap beautiful growth, plant friend? Homes, jobs, relationships? Can you find gratitude for having pruned something even if the choice was painful? What or who needs to be pruned away from your life? Negative thought patterns, assumptions, jealousy, bad haircuts?

Take 5 with your plants and explore these prompts:

- What is draining your soul right now? What conversations, tasks, or interactions are you avoiding? When you wake up in the morning or consider your upcoming week, what causes you stress or fear?

- Based on your answer to the question above, reflect on what isn't serving you. What might need to be pruned back? It might not be possible to simply snip the energy suckers out of your life, but brainstorm ways that you can change your attitude or approach in order to limit the energy that you spend on them.

- What has been pruned away in the past—it could be opportunities you missed, things taken from you, or things you deliberately chose to release—and what new growth came from it? How can those experiences speak into your current life experience?

Don't Cry over a Rotten Tomato

Of all the lessons I learned from my balcony garden, this is my favorite to share.

Some backstory: In 2017 my partner Billy and I had just moved in with each other after being long-distance for three years. We signed a lease on a tiny apartment with an even tinier nine-square-foot Juliet balcony. It was teensy but it was ours, and we were eager to settle into our new home together. Our first efforts to nest revolved around trying to grow some herbs and vegetables together, including a tiny tomato plant. We were both fiercely independent people, and this little garden was one of the first joint hobbies that we enjoyed together.

Pro tip: If your partner is struggling to come to terms with your love of houseplants, find a way to get them engaged with a type of plant or plant care that interests them. I found that it was easier for Billy to connect with growing edible plants that served a functional purpose than to appreciate my burgeoning collection of inedible houseplants. Growing this garden gave us common ground and allowed us to enjoy the process of nurturing something together. Once we established that, the rest was history (cut to our living in five hundred square feet with 160 houseplants not

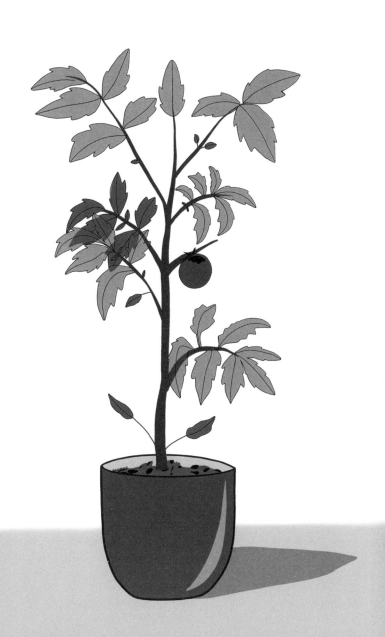

much later). I now jokingly advise couples to "start with a plant, then get a dog, then have a baby."

Our balcony garden came with new, shared responsibilities. We became a team committed to helping this little plant grow. We would text each other asking, "Did you water the tomato plant today?" or "Love, did you notice that the tomato grew two inches!?! We are nailing this!" The practice of caring for this plant became a fun game. We would smell the leaves and marvel at the growth of the foliage, which quickly grew from a mere four inches tall to three towering feet. Most important, we dreamed about what we were going to do with all of the tomatoes we would soon be harvesting.

Sitting on our couch and looking through the window at the plant, we'd conspire together: Would we make delicious tomato sauce with our crop? Would we preserve some of the leftover tomatoes in jars like my Italian cousins do? Or maybe we would slice the tomatoes up with salt and have platters of caprese when we entertained? The options for our bountiful harvest were endless.

Despite our best efforts, our plans were slightly thwarted, because the enormous tomato plant grew only one tomato. Yes, one tomato. We'd put so much work into this plant and had dreamed about our bountiful harvest, but we suddenly found ourselves looking at a single tomato nestled in our bush of green, fragrant foliage. But, like the naïve, joyful young gardeners we were, we stayed positive. We went right on ahead and said, "You know what? If this is the only tomato on the whole plant, it's got to be special, right? I bet it will be the most delicious tomato ever." Our plans and dreams surrounding the harvest got smaller, but to us, they were still big.

Once again, arm in arm on our couch, we'd peek out the window and discuss the various options for our sole tomato. After much debate, we landed on slicing it very thin, sprinkling it with flaky sea salt, and some homegrown basil, and enjoying it on our rooftop with some prosecco. We'd look out the window at our ripening tomato baby and salivate thinking of the teensy feast ahead of us. This tomato had us giggling and smiling and dreaming together. We continued caring for the plant: watering, smelling the leaves, singing to it, delighting in more fruitless foliage, and nurturing our beloved, singular tomato.

One day while we were both at work, a huge windstorm blew in and knocked the helpless tomato plant over. Our sole tomato was knocked off its stem and was completely inedible by the time we found it. Two months of caring and nurturing for our Little Tomato Plant That Could, all gone. That was a tough day for our household. I'd be lying if I said I didn't cry. I shed an embarrassing amount of tears over that lost tomato. I felt like a failure and that all our hard work had been for nothing. I mourned all the time we'd spent watering and caring for this plant, only to see it go to waste. And the fact that I was sitting on my couch crying over a rotten tomato made me feel not only like a failure, but also like an insane person.

Then it hit me: I hadn't just spent months nurturing this little plant in hopes of a delicious reward. I'd spent months on that couch holding Billy's hand as we dreamed about future meals together. We'd spent months coordinating care for our plant, celebrating little wins, fashioning tomato stakes out of chopsticks, and reading blogs on garden care together—months of two independent people slowly inching toward a life of teamwork together.

The success of our first tomato plant had nothing to do with the actual tomato, its growth and ripening and ultimate harvest—or lack of harvest. It had everything to do with the experience of growing the tomato together, what we learned about gardening for our future gardening seasons, and what we learned about each other through the process.

My fondest memories of that summer are of us cuddled up on the couch, dreaming about what to do with our (ultimately singular) bounty, and, for the first time, watching a plant grow. Witnessing this tiny seedling develop into a large, luscious plant, and watching a small yellow flower develop into a juicy red tomato, helped me understand the cycle of life in a deeper way. It was my first year trying to grow food, and there was so much to learn. It gave me great respect for the farmers of our country, who work hard to nurture plants on a large scale so we can afford the luxury of not understanding these processes.

Seeing that life cycle up close helped me to understand how fleeting life can be, and to treasure the present moment a little more, because I realized that the end result doesn't really matter. Although we didn't harvest any tomatoes that year, we harvested knowledge, connection, and teamwork.

it's not about the tomato.

That gardening season was many years ago, and to this day I still coach myself on life's little struggles, occasionally saying, "Maria, **it's not about the tomato**." It's become a little key I use to unlock that helpful sense of perspective when I get stressed out and overwhelmed thinking about the future. It's just simply . . . not about the "tomato" of whatever I'm being impatient about. When I was an unemployed actress desperately waiting to book my next job, I'd take a deep breath and hum, "It's not about the tomato." When I finally booked a show and had opening-night nerves, I repeated "It's not about the tomato," walking to the theater before the first performance. When I was patiently waiting for a marriage proposal in the sixth year of dating Billy . . . I'd use that phrase a LOT. As Billy and I currently save to buy our first home, I return to this mantra and know it will continue to serve me in every season of life.

Dig Deep

What's your tomato?

What about you, plant friend? Take 5 and find a quiet, plant-filled place to reflect and work through this exercise.

- What have you been nurturing in your life? Maybe it's a relationship, your career, a long-held dream. What's the thing you daydream

about, work toward, and long for? Write down
one or two "tomatoes," whether they're big or
small.

- Reflect on how that goal has been going. Do
you feel like you're making progress, or does
your goal feel distant? When you think about
your tomatoes, are you eager and excited
or anxious and stressed? Write down your
reactions.

- Take your eyes off the "tomato" for a moment,
plant friend. Marvel at exactly where you are.
Chances are, you're currently surrounded by
things that you only used to dream about
having. Maybe you always wanted to live
in this city you now reside in, maybe you
dreamed for years about that college diploma
you now take for granted, or perhaps you've
been building friendships that are now life-
giving and sustaining. By all means, chase your
"tomatoes," but don't forget to appreciate the
process and to delight in where you are.

Tips for growing a tomato plant

I know we're talking about metaphorical tomatoes here . . .
but I can't *not* give you a few tips about growing actual tomatoes:

- **Help them find their light:** Tomatoes need LOTS of light. Six to eight hours of direct sunlight a day will set them up for success.

- **Go deep:** Unlike with most other plants, you want to plant the root ball deep into the ground. When planting, remove the bottom leaves and bury the first few inches of the stem along with the root ball. The small hairs on the tomato stalk are actually "adventitious roots," meaning that when planted underground they will grow and develop as part of the root system and help stabilize the plant.

- **Be consistent:** Tomatoes need consistent moisture at their root zone. Don't let them dry out, go too long without water, or stay overly wet. Consistently moist soil is their happy place.

- **Feed them—they're hungry:** Tomato plants use a lot of nutrients as they spend their resources to grow these delicious fruits, so make sure you are fertilizing throughout the season.

- **Show your support:** Use a stake, cage, or trellis to give your tomatoes something to grow up and lean on as they grow delicious, juicy (and heavy) fruits!

- **Say goodbye to suckers:** Suckers are leaves or shoots that grow in between the main stem and branches of the tomato. While they are basically harmless, many gardeners prune these off the plants to encourage airflow and reinvest energy into the main plant.

- **Give it a friend!** Plant tomato plants with basil nearby. Basil is known to ward off pests like aphids, whiteflies, and tomato hornworms that tend to love tomato plants. Also, it makes harvesting the perfect caprese salad very easy!

A Letter to My Pepper Plant Going into Transplant Shock

Dear Pepper,

Yesterday I took you out of your seedling pot and transplanted you into your final home: the five-gallon container you'll live in during the growing season on my sunny balcony. Today you aren't very happy with me. You are going through some transplant shock, which is understandable, sweet pepper baby. You've gone from a tiny little pot, just large enough to house you and your delicate roots comfortably, to a larger container, filled with new, unknown soil that feels vast and foreign.

You're currently sulking, mourning your lost home

with droopy leaves. I know this process is hard and uncomfortable right now, but I promise, if you trust me, you'll be so much happier in your new home. You had outgrown your current pot, and if you stayed, your roots would have toppled over each other and made you so unhappy.

Your new pot, with all of its delicious organic, nutrient-rich soil, has so much space for you to stretch and grow! Think of the possibilities! Think of all the nutrients you'll absorb so you can become big and strong! Think of all of the delicious peppers you'll produce if you let yourself expand to your fullest potential. You couldn't grow peppers that large and delicious if you stayed in your small seedling home. I know it's scary at first, but you'll love it if you give it a chance.

Let's make a deal: Give it a month. Explore your new space, lift your leaves back up to face the sun and soak it in, establish your roots in this new soil, and let's circle back. Once you've adjusted, we can talk about returning you to your old nursery pot, if you still want to go back. But I have a feeling you'll see the beautiful potential for growth ahead of you and want to stay put.

You've got this, and I'll be here to help the whole time.

Love,
Maria, your Plant Parent

Dig Deep

Have you ever felt like this pepper plant? Going through transition and fearful of the unknown? New pots or people or homes can be intimidating, but if you let yourself grow into them and have the courage to put down roots, they can reveal opportunities you'd never have been able to see or experience in your previous space. Let your fear of uncertainty transform into excitement about the potential and possibility of what is new.

Take 5 with your plants and your journal

- Write down areas of your life that feel uncomfortable or overwhelming because they are new or different. Whether it's diving into the dating game, assuming a new job title, or settling into a new home, we all feel fear when we step into the unknown—even when the change is something good.

- Come up with three ways you can lean into this time of transition and grow boldly instead of shrinking back. Remind yourself that transition is a process, not a single action. Have patience and know that you will grow into your new situation, whatever it may be.

Make More Plants, Grow More Joy

Don't Hate, Propagate

Oh my goodness gracious, great balls of fire, propagating plants is so fun and such a beautiful way to inspire curiosity. It will turn you into a giddy five-year-old, no matter what age your body might be. Watching a root grow out of nowhere is just plain freaking fun. The first time you propagate a plant in water and watch roots grow is the coolest experience! You'll feel such ownership over your new plant baby and will have learned about the process of growing on a much deeper level. Propagation for the win!

Propagation is your chance to take the plants you've already got and make more plants . . . for FREE. It's when you either grow a new plant from a seed *or* you make a "copy" of the plant by taking a cutting from a mother plant to make a new baby clone plant. It's a fun and affordable way to grow your plant collection and to experience your plants as living things.

Different plants require different methods of propagation. They can be very simple or extremely complicated.

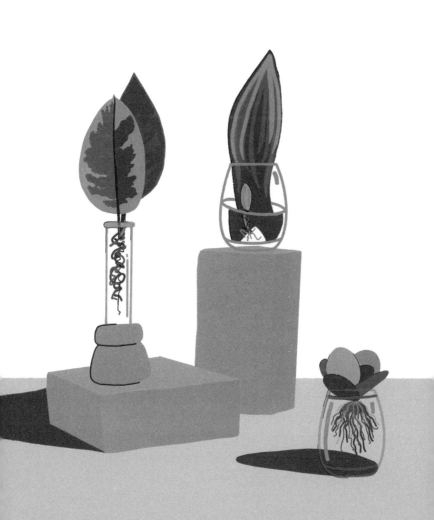

Most plants we know and love are propagated by seed or vegetative cutting. There are several different techniques when it comes to vegetative cuttings: stem tip cuttings, air layering, cane cuttings, whole leaf cuttings, leaf petiole cuttings, split-vein cuttings, even tissue culture. You can spend a lifetime experimenting with various propagation methods, cultivating curiosity and deepening your relationship to your plants and to life itself.

We're going to keep it simple here with two tried-and-true propagation methods for beginners. There are great resources at the back of this book to further develop your propagation skills. My advice is always to simply remain curious and to experiment.

How to Root Pothos Cuttings in Water

YOU'LL NEED:

- A sharp, sterile scissor or knife
- A glass of water
- A healthy, pest-free pothos plant (water-rooting also works well for other vining aroids such as *Philodendron* and *Monstera*)
- Rooting hormone (you don't absolutely need this if you don't have it, but it can help speed up the rooting process)

1. Find a nice long vine on your plant and locate the nodes. Nodes are the section of the plant

where new bud shoots and roots can grow. On your pothos or philodendron they will look like horizontal stripes that bulge a bit and have a little brown nub on the side. For some reason, I always think of them as the plant's knuckles. When cutting your vine off the mother plant, try and cut a nice long piece, three to four inches minimum, with several nodes to make several cuttings.

2. Take a stem tip cutting: Hold the section of vine you've cut and find the tip of it—meaning the end of the plant opposite from where you separated it from the mother plant. Locate the top two nodes. With your scissors, cut a quarter inch below the second node and remove the bottom leaf. Dip it in rooting hormone gel or a rooting hormone that can be used in water, if you have it, and pop that in your glass of water.

3. Take leaf bud cuttings with the remainder of your trimmed vine. Locate each node and snip it off the mother vine within a quarter inch on either side. Leave the leaf attached. Pop those in water. It's important to leave only a quarter inch of stem on either side of the node, as leaving more can cause them to rot. Compost the remainder of the stem.

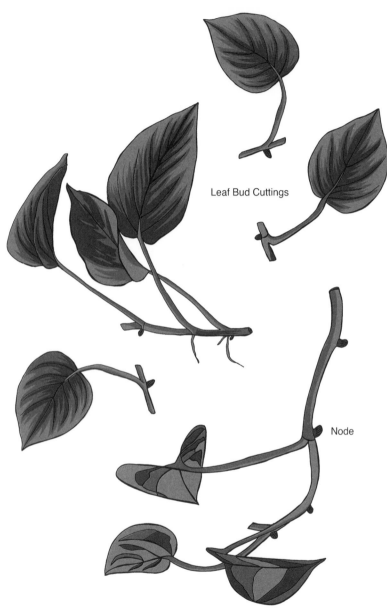

Leaf Bud Cuttings

Node

Stem Tip Cutting

4. Stick your glass of water and cuttings on your windowsill and watch what happens. Within a week or two you'll notice roots start to develop. Wait till the roots are two or three inches long and have started to branch before you transplant the cuttings into potting mix.

5. Once you have a nice, healthy, branching root system (called a root mat), pot your new cuttings in a small pot filled with high-quality potting mix.

6. Water your newly potted plant thoroughly.

7. Your plant will take a few weeks to establish in the soil, so don't be afraid if it doesn't look tremendously happy immediately after you've potted it up. Keep the soil a little moister than you normally would in these first few weeks, to help your new cutting adjust after going from pure water to potting mix.

8. Style your new plant in your home, or spread the plant love and gift it to one of your favorite people.

Tips for Water-Rooting a Plant

• Change the water every few days to keep it fresh.

- Don't wait too long to pot the cuttings in potting mix. The longer roots sit in water, the harder it will be for them to transition to growing media.

- If roots begin to rot (they will start to turn brown or black), trim them back and try again.

- Stay curious and have fun!

How to Root a Succulent Leaf

YOU'LL NEED:

- A sterile knife or scissor
- A succulent with lots of fleshy leaves, like an echeveria
- Potting mix
- A dish
- A misting bottle

1. Gently break or cut a leaf off of the succulent; you want to take the entire leaf as this is a whole leaf cutting, so make sure to break it off at the base of the leaf. Because this method doesn't have a 100 percent success rate, I suggest taking several leaves.

2. Put the leaf on a dish (make sure it's dry) to "cure." A callus will develop at the base of

the leaf where it was originally connected to the plant. This is crucial for the success of the propagation. The callus will look like a brown scab and will take several days to develop.

3. Once the leaves have cured, fill the dish with an airy, succulent potting mix that is slightly damp. Place the cured leaves on top of the potting mix. You can gently press them into the potting mix, but do not need to cover them with soil.

4. Be patient.

5. Slowly but surely, roots will start to burst out of the callus. Once they develop, start dampening the soil and roots with your spray bottle.

6. Like magic, the original leaf will start to slowly shrivel up and a new teensy tiny plantlet will grow. Once the mother leaf detaches, you can plant your new tiny succulent in a small pot. Stick it in a spot with nice, bright light and marvel at your new plant.

Although these instructions might feel high-maintenance or difficult, it's amazing how frequently this happens naturally in our plant collections. I have an heirloom jade plant, given to me by a friend; it was first gifted to her from a friend, and is probably twenty years old. As the plant continues to grow, leaves will fall off due to age or the occasional bump while getting moved around. I have found tiny plant-lets and shriveled leaves of this plant rooted in the soil of its own pot and the other pots around it on many occasions. The leaves go rogue and just propagate themselves without my help. It just goes to show that no matter how much we baby our plants, they are hardwired to survive and procreate, with or without us.

Share Your Cuttings

Keeping your cuttings is a great way to grow your collection, but sharing your cuttings is a great way to spread the planty love and bring joy to others. My favorite plants in my collection are those that were gifted to me as small cuttings and that have slowly grown into large plants. I not only enjoy the beauty of these plants, but I remember the stories behind them. If you do decide to share some cuttings, make sure they are disease- and pest-free before you gift them. Fun fact: some species of plants are patented and cannot be propagated without a license, so make sure you are propagating and gifting an unpatented plant. Swing by the "Growing Together" chapter for tips on connecting with others through plant swaps.

Get propagating, grow some joy, and share those cuttings to create a beautiful ripple effect of happiness and kindness throughout your planty community.

"SEEDS HAVE TOMORROW READY-BUILT INTO THEM."

—Dr. Sue Stuart Smith,
The Well-Gardened Mind

The Show of Seed Starting

Seeds symbolize not only a promise of growth to come, but also a responsibility to nurture whatever we are sowing. Their purpose in nature is reflected in our lives and our language. People talk about "planting the seed of an idea" or "sowing seeds of doubt." There is nothing more joyful than holding a dormant seed, putting it in the earth, and watching it burst forth with life.

Craig LeHoullier knew this joy. In an act of plant friend kindness, he sent me an envelope of micro-dwarf tomato seeds after I interviewed him on my podcast about his book *Epic Tomatoes*. In my tiny NYC apartment, with this small packet of seeds, I got a front-row seat to Mother Nature's longest-running show: germination. I was excited and slightly nervous to try starting these seeds, as I didn't want Craig's sweet gesture to be for nothing. But I was determined and knew that despite my lack of a garden shed, or any proper seed-starting equipment, *the show must go on.*

My first seed-starting experience can be likened to an extremely low-budget community theater production of *Guys and Dolls*: not the most visually appealing production, its success by no means assured, but performed with a whole lot of heart. The "germination station" was an upcycled plastic egg carton with holes I stabbed with a steak knife. After the seeds were tucked in the egg reservoirs with damp seed-starting mix, I wrapped the whole kit and kaboodle in plastic wrap, placed it on a heating pad that I usually only used for menstrual cramps, and said a prayer. These seeds were seasoned professionals. My low-budget setup didn't scare them.

Lo and behold, after a few cozy days on the heating pad, the opening number started: Tiny cotyledons pressed up against the plastic, cuing me to set them free. I transferred them to the bookshelf that I had outfitted with a grow light for my houseplants, and the show continued.

The dance my seedlings were able to perform despite being underwatered was remarkable. They could be completely wilted, lying limp on the soil, and a drink of water would swiftly revive them to stand straight up and bask in the (artificial) sun. They were like circus contortionists. I shouldn't admit this, but I might have sometimes waited a little too long to water them just to enjoy an encore. The plot unfolded day by day: one set of true leaves, then another. Soon the intoxicating, delicious perfume of tomato leaves filled my bedroom.

At this point I was hooked. I visited my plants every day, checking on their growth and beaming with pride at what I'd grown in my tiny space. Back then I was naïve enough to think that I had something to do with these seeds' preprogrammed ability to flourish. I know better now. It was their natural talent.

Soon these green entertainers were ready for the big time—not Broadway, but my balcony. Lined up in a row like Rockettes, these sweet plants hit their stride in the sun's spotlight. They were triple threats: growing gorgeous green leaves, smelling amazing, and even flowering. In the fall, the plants withered and returned to the soil, spreading their seeds in the fruit we didn't harvest and creating opportunities for germination for an encore performance the following year. Experiencing that full life cycle was the delight of my summer—a smash hit.

Start Seeds, Spark Joy

Gift yourself tickets to this stellar performance for the cost of a ninety-nine-cent seed packet. Choose a plant you are curious about, read the instructions for planting, and get growing.

Dig Deep

You are an ever-evolving, ever-changing garden, plant friend. You have a great variety of "seeds" within you; their germination, growth, and life cycles are all different, but they're all perfectly timed in the scope of your life. Some are annuals, some perennials; some are grown for beauty, some for function; some invite pests, some won't make it, and some will thrive beyond your wildest imagination. Seeds of success, joy, and love are waiting to germinate at the exact right time they were destined to.

Take 5 with your plants and reflect on the "seeds" of your life: your career, relationships, friendships, mental or physical health. Pick one area of potential growth to focus on, and consider:

- What is your vision for this "seed"? What will it grow up into? Define what success looks like so you know what you're growing toward.

- Seeds take time to grow! Some can shoot up overnight and some pop only after a long period of time. What are you impatient about right now? Can you reframe your anxiety and lean into the fact that everything is happening exactly how it should be?

- How can you nurture this area of potential— perhaps like you would dote on a seedling, with water, sunlight, and love? Come up with three active steps you can take to get yourself closer to where you'd like to be.

The Power of Flowers

One of the most meaningful gifts I ever received was a handpicked bouquet of wildflowers from Billy, on our first scheduled wedding day. After becoming engaged in 2019, we were very excited to get married in September 2020. The COVID-19 pandemic had other plans, and we were forced to reschedule. The decision to postpone was stressful, and that season of life was filled with lots of tears and fear around what to do about "our big day."

On our original wedding date, Billy and I rented a cottage on a remote island in Maine, to be alone and allow space for whatever feelings bubbled up. We decided to have a commitment ceremony on the beach, just the two of us, to honor our original plans. Before the "ceremony," Billy left for a few minutes and returned with a vibrant bouquet of wildflowers and greenery he had foraged around the island. It was far more beautiful than any bouquet I could have ordered from a florist, because it was made by him, for me, with love.

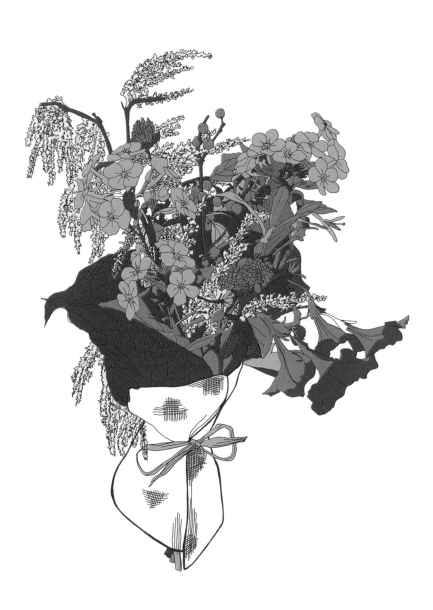

As we stood barefoot in the sand, making promises to each other in our makeshift ceremony, I held the bouquet, wrapped in a cloth napkin from our cabin. It was a sweet, simple gift from him, but also a symbol that formalized our vow exchange. Even if we had no officiant, no wedding dress, and our loved ones were miles away, the blooms gave me that whimsical bridal feel every woman thinks about when she imagines getting married. I'm thankful for that handful of blooms that gave me permission to feel like a bride, even if I couldn't have the wedding I'd imagined.

Flowers make people happy. We are just hardwired to love them. Maybe it's because, from an evolutionary standpoint, we'd see a flower and know it would develop into something edible, or that the sweet honey made by its pollinators must be nearby. Whatever our known or unknown bias is, flowers are little joy bombs just waiting to be cut or grown. We've been cultivating flowers for more than five thousand years,[1] and the booming cut flower industry is proof in itself that humans continue to use flowers to bring joy to their lives and even to communicate with others. We send bouquets of congratulations, sympathy, and "just because," and live for the moment our orchid or African violet shows signs of blooming. Sigmund Freud, an orchid lover,[2] said, "The enjoyment of beauty has a peculiar, mildly intoxicating quality of feeling. Beauty has no obvious use; nor is there any clear cultural necessity for it. Yet civilization could not do without it." Agreed.

If you want to cultivate more joy in your life, flowers are a great way to do so. Get bloomin', baby.

Ways to Grow Joy with Flowers

Support your local florist, grocer, or farmers market vendor by purchasing a bouquet of in-season flowers

A small posy will make any room feel fresh and bring a smile to your face. Developing a relationship with your local florist is also a wonderful way to grow deeper roots in your community. When I lived in Long Island City, I befriended my local florists (shout-out to the guys at fLorEsta in LIC), who turned out to be wonderful sources of knowledge in my plant parenthood journey. They taught me about drainage and the importance of high-quality potting mix, and indulged my succulent-collecting obsession when I was first starting off.

One day I went by to purchase some succulents, and the owner sent me home with a bud vase with a single flower in it as a gift. Once the flower faded, I went back to buy another one to replace it. I got into the habit of visiting the shop on my way home from the subway to see what beautiful flowers were in season that I could pop into that bud vase. Since I was buying only one flower at a time, this was an extremely affordable treat, often cheaper than a latté from my local coffee shop, and the bloom would bring me joy all week long as it sat cheerfully on my kitchen counter.

Gift a bouquet to a friend

We know the happiness that keeping flowers in your home can bring, so why not spread the plant love and gift an unexpecting friend a bouquet to brighten their day? She'll think of you every time she looks at her little vase of sunshine. Try adding a note to your "just because" bouquet and share a silly memory, something you appreciate about her or even a line of poetry.

Grow houseplants that bloom!

Orchids, African violets, and hoya are a great place to start. *Hoya* is an amazing genus, with over two hundred different species of plants, each with unique flowers in a variety of shapes, colors, and scents. Hoya are commonly referred to as porcelain or wax plant, as their shiny flowers appear wax-like and almost unreal. African violets are another fantastic option for plants that bloom indoors. I inherited an African violet from a friend that withheld its blooms from me for over a year. The day that I saw the cluster of buds in the center of its fuzzy leaves, I got so excited I thought my head would explode. The plant then gifted us with the most gorgeous bouquet of silvery purple blooms, and it has rebloomed for us many times.

Never knowing when the blooms will come is a fun exercise in anticipation, and the stunning payoff is always worth the wait. Orchids have it all: gorgeous flowers of all shapes, sizes, and colors, intoxicating scents found in many perfumes, and beautiful foliage with wacky roots that are delightful, even when the plant isn't in bloom. Orchids are a great choice for the Curious Collector Plant Parent, which you'll learn about in a little bit. I have wonderful 101 care guides for hoya, African violets, and orchids on the *Bloom and Grow Radio* Podcast if you feel inspired to experiment with growing them![3]

Grow bulbs indoors to beat winter blues

Winter can be a real bummer. Days are shorter, there's less light, motivation wanes, and many of our foliage houseplants' growth slows, while some even lose leaves and go dormant. For plant parents who live to see growth and blooms, it's easy to feel stagnant in the winter months. Growing bulbs indoors is, hands down, the best winter blues buster I've ever experienced. I live for the moment potted amaryllises hit grocery stores across the country before the holidays. I love setting up paperwhites in see-through vases to watch both their roots and shoots go through rapid expansion.

For a quick "hit" of springtime in the midst of the slow season, bulbs are the answer. Some bulbs require cold periods to develop flower buds, which can get a bit confusing and high-maintenance for beginners. If you're a first-time bulb grower, I recommend picking up a potted amaryllis, paperwhite, or hyacinth that is already growing. You can find these familiar potted plants at your grocery store, garden center, or florist next time they are in season. Look for potted or water-rooted bulbs that are already developing flower buds but haven't opened yet.

Although it's hard to resist picking the gorgeous blooming pots at the store, you want to be able to experience the entire life cycle of the flower, and choosing the yet-to-bloom pots will give you the longest, most joyful ride. You can also negotiate with yourself and choose one that has several shoots in different states of blooming—which is a metaphor for life itself, isn't it?

Dig Deep

One of the reasons flowers are such beautiful additions to our lives is that they hold beauty at every stage of their development. We all love the glory of a flower in its prime, but the buds, with their hints of color, and the almost-spent flowers, with their loose, artfully drooping petals, are lovely in their own right.

Take 5 with your plants and reflect on how you can appreciate every stage of "bloom" in your life—from the tightly furled buds of possibility, to the joyful colors of fully realized dreams, to the chaotic beauty of good things that have begun to fade away.

Plants + The Home

Our homes are full of inanimate objects: furniture, electronics, clothes in closets. Over time, our sacred spaces can start to feel stale and uninspiring. Plants are a great solution to this problem, as they bring ever-changing life to our space and give us the opportunity to be reminded of growth on a daily basis.

Nothing illustrates the importance of bringing plants indoors to freshen things up more than Biophilic design.

Biophilia and Biophilic Design

The concept of Biophilia is one of the pillars of the plant/person connection, popularized by E. O. Wilson, a Harvard entomologist, in the 1980s but first introduced by psychologist Erich Fromm in the '70s. Fromm described it as "the passionate love of life and of all that is alive." Wilson defines Biophilia as "the innately emotional affiliation of human beings to other living organisms."

I'm sold. Think about it: We ourselves are living, so we instinctively relate to other living things. Beyond that, humans were created and evolved in nature. We are hardwired to be at ease in natural settings. Years of technology usage and urban living might have left us a bit disconnected from it, but plant friend, the instinct is there, within you. There is a reason we feel that full-body, head-to-toe rush of relaxation as we hear a babbling brook or crackling fire, or when we're surrounded by lush green vegetation. It's Biophilia. It's awesome.

Start paying attention to the way you feel when you're in nature, or spending time with your plants, and you'll be sold too.

Biophilic Design is a way of incorporating the natural world into our indoor spaces. It takes the concept of Biophilia one step further by acknowledging this intrinsic connection between humans and nature and the immense benefit humans reap when this connection is considered in the design of spaces we inhabit. We aren't just talking about putting out adorable pillows with plants printed on them, but also considering the lines of a building, what direction the windows face, the materials used to construct the building, and much more, all in order to create the best opportunity for the people inside to experience the benefits of being outside.

I am forever thankful to Terrapin Bright Green, LLC, for publishing *14 Principles of Biophilic Design*, an unbelievably comprehensive breakdown of all things Biophilic Design, on all scales. Since reading the report, I've come to look at every corner in every room of my home as an opportunity to merge outdoor and indoor.

Once I began applying these principles in my home, my stuffy home office full of glowing screens and windowless walls turned into a planty retreat with a living green wall, natural wooden desk, a pair of snake plants (*Dracaena* spp.) flanking my computer monitor, and a playlist of nature sounds underscoring my workday. My bedroom is now a restorative oasis, with plants surrounding my bed to allow me to wake up to a jungle of Monstera leaves instead of to the glow of my phone. My kitchen has fresh herbs growing in it, so that I can engage all of my senses in preparing and connecting with my food and drink: from picking the mint, to breathing in its crisp scent, to blending it into my green smoothie or mixing it into a mojito.

Now that so many studies are proving that Biophilic Design in office spaces can decrease stress and increase employee well-being, we see inspirational buildings such as Amazon's Seattle Spheres. These life-sized terrariums, filled with over forty thousand plants, are a haven for employees to work, have meetings, and take restorative breaks in. I was lucky enough to visit the Spheres, and the overwhelming sense of delight that envelops you when you walk inside is hard to describe. Singapore can boast that almost 50 percent of the seven-hundred-square-kilometer city is "under green cover."[1] It's also home to the Parkroyal Collection on Pickering, a concept hotel whose "hotel in a garden" exterior looks like a tropical oasis.

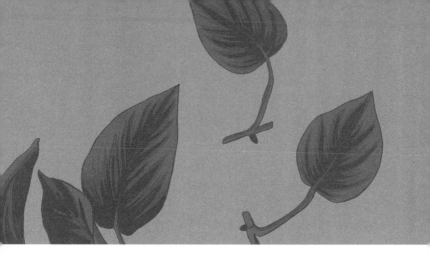

PLANTS CAN BE

FANTASTIC
COWORKERS

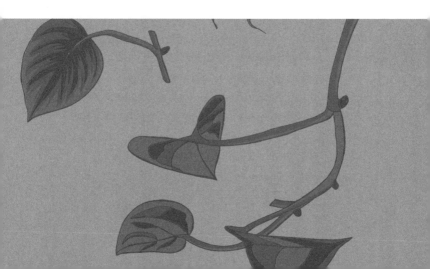

The concepts of Biophilic Design can be applied on any scale: from a small home office to an entire office building. Let's talk about how you can use these concepts in two practical ways—in your office and in your home—to cultivate more joy throughout your day.

Bring Plants into Your Workspace

The workplace is where we will experience the majority of our stress and spend most of our time. So let's use plants to decrease stress and increase happiness throughout our workdays, whether your workplace is a teensy corner in your apartment or a traditional corner office with a view.

Plants can be fantastic coworkers: They are always available to listen or take a break with, and they never give you passive-aggressive sass. Whether or not you commute to an office, you're likely spending much of your day (up to eleven hours) at a screen, which is a no-no when it comes to cultivating joy throughout your workday.

A global study[2] reports that workers in environments with natural elements such as greenery and sunlight benefit from a 15 percent higher level of well-being, a 6 percent increase in productivity, and a 15 percent increase in creativity! Wowza. The top five elements workers desire in an office are, in order: natural light, indoor plants, a quiet working space, a view of the sea, and bright colors. I bet you

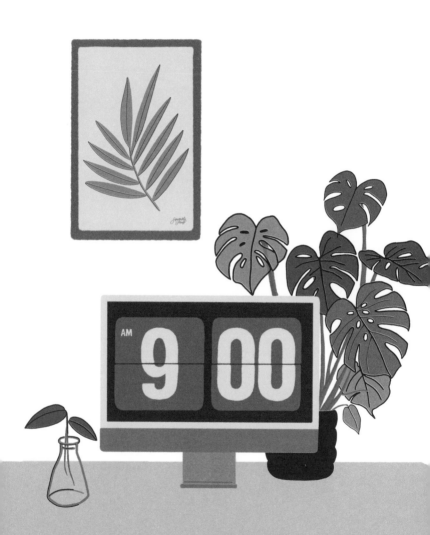

can uplevel at least one of these elements in your current work setup.

Tips for growing joy in your office greenspace

1. **Have plants in your sight line.** It's that simple. Make it so no matter where you turn your head, you see a green friend, waving at you with its leaves, cheering you on through your back-to-back meetings and deadlines. I have plants beside my computer monitor and plants on the bookshelf behind me, which make a killer video conferencing background. This means I can experience nature throughout my workday and have lots of reminders to take a screen break and engage with plants.

2. **Take micro screen breaks with plants.** If you are one of the nearly two-thirds of Americans who report having digital eye strain, doctors recommend, in addition to using larger screens and fonts, taking forty-second screen breaks every twenty minutes. Spend forty seconds looking at objects that are far away from you, ideally twenty feet, to let your eyes rest from looking directly at your screen all day.[3] If you can't see twenty feet in front of you in your office, keep a plant with a pretty

leaf pattern across the room, so you can disconnect from your screen and let your eyes take in the beautiful, natural pattern during your micro break.

3. **Push your desk up against a window.** The easiest way to connect with nature while indoors is to simply look at it.[4] Positioning your desk up against a window with a view of nature allows your eyes to rest by focusing on trees at different distances, and more important, gives you an opportunity to spy on people in the park nearby. In Biophilic Design, there is a concept called "non-rhythmic sensory stimuli," similar to those beautiful moments of fascination and involuntary attention we talked about earlier, that basically means it feels good to have random, unpredictable things happen around you, like clouds passing by, plant life rustling, or insects moving. This is hard to replicate indoors, but by pushing your desk up against a window, you have the opportunity to experience weather changes, pollinators floating from flower to flower in your window box, and the beauty of wind rustling through nearby trees.

   - If you work from home and are able to, setting up a bird feeder outside your office window is a wonderful way to allow your local birds to surprise and delight you with their flights, funny behavior, and song all throughout your workday.

4. **Utilize your vertical space.** Most offices, whether work-from-home setups or standard cubicles, don't have a lot of floor or desk space up for grabs. To bring plants into your space without giving up valuable desk space, hang plants on the walls or in your windows, or even install grow lights (you can purchase frames with grow lights built into them) to make your plants look like art around you. Check out the resources at the end of the book for some recommended hanging planters and products.

5. **Listen to nature.** Remember all the tips from the "Engage Your Senses" chapter? Apply them here! Underscore your workday with sounds of your favorite nature scenes, whether it's waves crashing on a beach or a storm in the rain forest. If you can, set up a small water feature so you can enjoy the relaxing sound of trickling water and feel like you're in the forest while meeting your next deadline.

6. **Sniff transcendent scents.** Diffuse botanical oils in your office for constant forest vibes or for a mid-afternoon pick-me-up. I have a

rotation of hinoki, lavender, and eucalyptus and mix and match them depending on the mood I'm in at the beginning of my workday.

7. **Nonliving nature.** If living plants that require water and soil near your expensive computer isn't your thing, I totally get it. Although I always suggest prioritizing the real thing over the fake thing, fake plants are better than nothing. Even if you can't have plants, you can reap the emotional and cognitive benefits from other aspects of Biophilic Design.

   a. Here are some nonliving ideas for your workspace:

      i. Art that represents nature, plants, or an outdoor location that relaxes you

      ii. Botanical prints or wallpaper

      iii. Detailed pictures of the forest or natural scenes that you can zone off into

      iv. An enclosed terrarium of a scene that makes you smile

      v. A desk made out of natural material like wood or stone

      vi. Dried grasses or flowers in a vase

8. **Take restorative breaks.** Use the skills you learned in the "Take 5" sections of the book

and apply them throughout the workday.
Set a timer on your phone for a reminder to
engage with nature once an hour. Whether it's
taking a quick screen break to look at a plant
or to gaze through your window, wiping dust
off leaves, smelling an essential oil, taking
a quick walk outside, or tending to a plant,
give yourself a break to stretch, refocus, and
practice presence with your plants to find
more mindfulness in your day.

Note: Make sure you pick plants that work for your office lighting environment. Visit the appendix at the end of this book to learn more.

Create Your Planty Restorative Nook

Okay, plant friend, it's time to create your restorative nook. Here's where everything we've learned so far comes together in a beautifully planty bow. This is where you can apply *Growing Joy* practices to bring some evergreen stillness and delight to your life by strategically designing an area of your home with plants.

A restorative nook is a place where you can disconnect from screens and busyness and reconnect with yourself by surrounding yourself with plants. Your nook is a sacred place to reset, realign, and step away from the never-ending stressors of daily life and to-do lists. Everyone's restorative nooks will look different depending on their aesthetic, home size, plant collection, and lifestyle, but whether it's a small corner or an entire room, carving out an area to claim as your own and dedicate to intentional and restorative living can be a total game changer.

In Attention Restoration, the Kaplans talk about four components of the environment that are great inspirations when thinking about the restorative space you want to create. Below I've quoted their original concepts and suggested a few ideas for how to translate them into your personal space.

"Being away: being distinctly removed, either physically or conceptually, from the everyday environment."

- Where in your home might you be able to carve out a little nook for yourself? Locate a room, or even a corner, that you can claim as your own. Maybe it's a comfy chair in the corner of your bedroom, a part of your basement bedecked with grow lights, or an unused guest room. Your nook could also be outside your home, perhaps on a balcony or in your backyard. Get creative!

- No space? No problem. Listen, not everyone has space in a home to dedicate to this work. I get it. So let's try it in miniature! Create a restorative world in a terrarium that can transport you every time you peer inside. Keep it on your desk, or wherever you want to create a place of peace and whimsy. Allow yourself to let your imagination run free within the confines of that small glass vessel. You can choose whatever style of scene you'd like, whether it be a tiny forest, a desertscape, or a beach, and choose plants accordingly. Check out the resources in the back of this book for terrarium guides.[5]

"Fascination: containing patterns that hold one's attention effortlessly."

- As you design your nook, incorporate elements of nature that you can get lost in. Choose a variety of plants with interesting leaf patterns to keep you engaged. Add photographs of fractals or feature a window with a view of nature, so you can watch birds or other pollinators fly by.

- Mix it up! Another way to encourage fascination is by mixing up your nook's look. Instead of its being a static location, think of your nook as an evolving and growing space. Try switching plants around, changing the way you've styled them, or putting different art in your frames. One approachable way to do this is by changing your space with the natural rhythm of the seasons—that way your space will always feel visually interesting.

"Extent: having scope and coherence that allow one to remain engaged."

- This can be tricky, because you can't just fill your home with a thousand plants. Try and design your restorative space to have several different elements to keep the space engaging over a long period of time.

"Compatibility: fitting with and supporting what one wants or is inclined to do."[6]

- "Compatibility" is key to cultivating joy with plants. Some people find the most joy watching tomato plants go from flower to fruit in their gardens; others revel in the rare and unusual aroids that give a prehistoric, jungle vibe to any home. Some simply want plants they can take pride in not killing. It's simple: Pick plants that you love, and surround yourself with them!

Using these four pillars of a restorative space, think about what natural things you are drawn to and dream about your ideal environment.

Tips for building your restorative, planty environment

- Go screen-free. Try your best to leave your phones, screens, and distractions away from this sacred space. Treat your restorative nook as a sanctuary. This will train you to get into a relaxed mindset the minute you enter it and help create that transportive "away from it all" experience that we normally reserve for vacations with piña coladas.

- Make sure you have a comfortable seat to allow yourself to kick back and relax amidst your green friends.

- Use a variety of different types of plants in your space so you can enjoy the different patterns on their leaves. Let your eyes drift across the space and land on different leaf patterns and shapes and invite "soft fascination" to wash over you. You will be shocked at how good it feels to give yourself the space to simply zone out on a plant leaf while tracing the pattern with your eyes or observing how light moves across a leaf.

- Play your favorite music or try some nature soundtracks.

- Choose colors and textures you love. From a Biophilic Design perspective, earth tones will keep you "zenned out." But choosing color can be very personal, so if you love bright colors and they make you happy, go for it!

Your space and what you find restorative will change, and that's okay

However you design your space and whatever limitations you have, try your best to surround yourself with plants that bring you joy in that moment. Your space will change and grow as you change and grow. I've had three homes since I've taken up this plant care hobby, and my restorative spaces have looked different in every single one based on the confines of the space and my tastes at that moment in time—everything from my first tiny balcony to the plant filled loft I wrote this book in.

Other options for your restorative space

- An area in your bedroom
- A corner of your couch
- A balcony or patio (for you lucky ducks who live in a place where you can keep plants outdoors year-round)
- An unused area in your basement or attic
- A garden

Ways to unwind in your restorative space

- Keep a gratitude journal.
- Play your favorite music.
- Call your best friend (this breaks the no-screen rule, but connecting with people you love is a fine exception).
- Write to your intuition:
  - Ask a question about something that's been bothering you.
  - Take three deep breaths and allow your mind to clear, put pen to paper, and write, stream of consciousness with no judgment.
  - After you are finished writing, write "Why?"
  - Take three more breaths and allow yourself to respond.
  - After you've finished responding, write "Why?" again and continue this process, going deeper and deeper as you coach yourself through your struggles. Opening a dialogue within yourself can be unnerving, but it's a beautiful way to cultivate a deeper relationship with your true self.

- Read a book. *The Overstory* by Richard Powers will change the way you see trees and humanity.

- Read poetry. Ross Gay is my favorite planty poet; he writes all about gardens and life. I like to say "A poem a day by Ross Gay keeps the blues away."

- Meditate. Do the breathing practices from the "Take 5" section, use a meditation app, or try some breathing exercises—however you want to bring space and stillness to your mind, go for it.

- Invite a friend to come over and have a good laugh or deep conversation. Try and stay off your screens and dive deep to enjoy the true joy a good friendship brings.

Create a lush jungle oasis in your bathroom!

I have had a bathroom with a window on my vision board since I first began caring for plants. Only New Yorkers understand the true plight of never having bathrooms with a window. It seems like a natural thing to have . . . but not in NYC. There is something so appealing about filling your bathroom with plants and enjoying them as you shower. If you are a bath taker, adding lush plants to your bathtub surroundings is an easy way to add restorative jungle vibes to your bath-time routine.

If you don't have a window in your bathroom, take inspiration from my friend Darryl Cheng, author of *The New Plant Parent*, who has "hacked" his way into his jungle oasis bathroom retreat. Darryl set up grow lights on timers, which run through the night while he is asleep to keep his plants happy (and provide a great night-light for midnight bathroom breaks). Note: Using grow lights in bathrooms can be dangerous, so make sure you read your manual and organize wiring away from any water sources.

Know Yourself, Grow Yourself

What Is Your Plant Parent Personality?

To grow joy and not stress when it comes to plant care, you've got to make your plant collection work for you. One of the most frequent questions I get asked is "What is the best starter plant for a beginner?" My answer is: "There's no such thing." Just as there isn't the right starter pet for everyone, I don't believe there's a blanket "great starter plant." It's all about picking the right plant for your personality, environment, and lifestyle.

Back in my plant-killer days, I brought home the wrong plants for my space and lifestyle, and proceeded to kill them all because they didn't work for me. My plant-killer tendencies were a source of embarrassment and stress—the exact opposite of joy. In order to change that dynamic, I had to speed-date different types of plants until I found the ones that worked for my home and helped reduce my daily stress levels, instead of increasing them.

As a lover of personality tests I've always been fascinated by personality archetypes and how they manifest in different people. Over my years of podcasting about plant care, I've interacted with thousands of listeners across the world and noticed distinct personality archetypes that correspond with different lifestyles. I created the Plant Parent Personality Quiz on my website to help everyone accurately assess what kind of plant person they are and to direct them to curated lists of the right plants, DIY projects, and free educational resources that are tailor-made for them.

Here is an overview of each personality. Read them all, see what resonates, and integrate those lessons into your life! If you want to dive deeper and unlock your plant parent potential, plus get a longer list of recommended plants and free educational resources, find your official personality type for free at bloomandgrowradio.com/personality.

Mindful Plant Parent

If you're a Mindful Plant Parent, you'll be all in on the *Growing Joy* practices from page one! You love to engage with your plants on a daily basis, with the intention of increasing presence and mindfulness in your daily life. Whether it's incorporating plants into your morning routine, using them during your midday meditations, or unwinding with them in the evening, you're open and ready.

You rock at: consistency, making space and time to engage with your plants, and eagerly learning every lesson a plant can teach you

You might struggle with: overwatering. Because you love to care for your plants, you are prone to *overloving* them. When you engage with your plants daily, it's easy to grab the watering can to feel like you're helping them, but very few plants require daily watering. Make sure you keep your plants in a light, airy potting mix with lots of drainage. Understand their care requirements and stick to them. Never prioritize your desire to nurture over the plant's care requirements. There are plenty of ways to engage with your plants *without* watering them, so stick with those and you'll be golden.

Try these plants: Any type of moisture-loving plant will be your friend, because it will be ready for more TLC than plants that require periods of drought. Try orchids, ferns, prayer plants (Marantaceae family), African violets, herbs, begonias, or air plants (*Tillandsia* spp).

Make Sure to Try These *Growing Joy* Practices

- Look at the list of ways to engage with your plants besides watering in the "Rooted in Routine" chapter (see page 13).

- Play around with every exercise in the "Plant Seeds of Delight" chapter (see page 86) to further your mindfulness and connection to your living green friends.

- Because you are so connected to your plant collection, losing a plant might be tough. When and if that happens, make sure you read the "On Plant Death" section (see page 173).

Low-Key Plant Parent

You wake up to seize the day and are usually juggling a million things like a boss. You love having plants in your home, but don't have a ton of time to devote to plant care. You appreciate plants as living decorative pieces in your home. You love to have them in your space to help you relax and reconnect with nature in the rare moments you have to pause and unwind, but you need a low-maintenance plant care routine that won't have you stressing over your schedule.

You rock at: appreciating the joy plants can bring to your home, and giving your plants the time and space they need to grow at their own pace

You might struggle with: forgetting your plant care routine and underwatering a plant or two in certain seasons of life. It might help to set weekly and monthly reminders for yourself to check in on your plants and make sure they are watered and happy.

Try these plants: Low-maintenance, drought-tolerant plants are going to be your besties. You might also try using passive hydroponic setups or self-watering planters. Try snake plants, Haworthias, ZZ plant, hoya, or a corn plant.

Make Sure to Try These *Growing Joy* Practices:

- Schedule some plant-based self-care time into your calendar. Once it's on your calendar, commit to making it happen! Give Forest Bathing a try (see page 40), and leave your to-do list and electronics behind to truly connect with nature and have some "you time." If you travel a lot, try and make time to visit local parks and botanical gardens to reap the benefits of being with plants even when you're not at home.

- Try a hydroponic setup for your plants (see page 77).

- Visit the "Plants + The Home" chapter (see page 137) for lots of fun ways to incorporate plant-inspired décor into your space without even needing to use living plants.

Curious Collector
Plant Parent

For you, plants are like Pokémon: You gotta catch 'em all. We can find you nestled in your indoor jungle of rare and wacky plants, scouring the Web for the sexiest, most sought-after, most photo-ready plants. No plant is too weird, too rare, or too expensive (within reason) for you to try! You are constantly looking for ways to become a better plant parent: by experimenting with different growing mediums, pots, watering techniques, and families of plants to see which ones thrive best in your home. You love to bring new plants into your space and nurture them. You're super proud of your incredibly varied and unique collection.

You rock at: experimenting, remaining curious, and learning about the wild world of plants

You might struggle with: growing your collection at a healthy, sustainable rate. Be careful not to overwhelm yourself with too many new plants at once. Focus on introducing plants at a steady pace. Make sure you know how to care for the plant friends you already have before you bring more in!

Try these plants: **Take a deep dive into collecting different species from one genus such as *Hoya*, *Philodendron*, or *Calathea*.**

Make Sure to Try These *Growing Joy* Practices:

- The heart-shaped leaf practice (see page 55) could be a very fun inspiration for an entire plant collection dedicated to heart-shaped foliage.

- Experiment with collecting plants that bloom (see page 134) to keep your collection diversified with pops of colorful flowers amidst your green foliage.

- One of the best ways to learn more about the wide world of plants is by connecting with the plant community. Try growing some planty friendships (see page 190).

- If your collecting ever tips from joyful to overwhelming, consider a plant pause (see page 180).

Design-Based Plant Parent

We can find you in your gorgeously curated home filled with pieces (living and inanimate) that you adore. You use plants to elevate your space, because you feel plants bring life and joy to a home. The structural elements of their leaves and blooms are what draw you to them, and you find all of the living patterns mesmerizing. You are up to speed on all the design trends and love using plants as vehicles to achieve your greatest design dreams.

You rock at: harnessing your innate creativity to curate a beautiful home filled with gorgeous plants. Your eye for design rivals any magazine's or blog's and helps you see combinations of plants and décor pieces that the average person wouldn't be able to visualize.

You might struggle with: putting the plant's needs above your design needs. It's important to design a beautiful home, but a plant's lighting and care requirements will ultimately determine where it will thrive in your home.

Try these plants: Plants with structural elements and beautiful leaf patterns are going to delight your inner designer. Try the friendship plant (*Pilea peperomioides*), fiddle leaf fig (*Ficus lyrata*), any type of *Monstera* (*M. adansonii, M. deliciosa*), Buddha belly (*Jatropha podagrica*), or a large gorgeous palm. Look for foliage variation and variegation with interesting colors and patterns that make your heart sing!

Make Sure to Try These *Growing Joy* Practices:

- Check out the "Plants + The Home" chapter for new design inspiration to create a nature-filled space.

- To make sure you understand your indoor lighting environment, swing by the "Understanding Light" section (see page 215).

- Play with mixing both foliage and flowers into your collection through cut flower bouquets (see page 133) and plants that flower (see page 134).

Urban Farmer Plant Parent

We can find you in the kitchen slicing into juicy homegrown tomatoes and cooking with the herbs you proudly tend to on your windowsill or balcony. You're using the space you have, whether it's an outdoor area or a grow light setup, to grow things you can cook, preserve, and drink. You think the best reward of growing something . . . is consuming it! Gardening is a daily practice, so you are very connected to your plants, especially throughout the growing season. You love feeling personally connected to the food you eat by watching it grow, and you find gardening to be the most relaxing and satisfying hobby. Store-bought tomatoes and lettuce will never taste the same after you grow them yourself.

You rock at: understanding the importance of connecting with the food on your plate. Friends are always asking for your recipes! You delight in nurturing your plants and watching them grow from seedlings.

You might struggle with: having the right conditions to grow food well. Herbs and veggies require six to eight hours of direct light for a great harvest, so you'll need some epic windows, an unobstructed balcony/porch/lawn, or some grow lights to get the best harvest.

Try these plants: if you have grow lights, pick whatever food you love eating and go for it. I love micro-dwarf tomato plants and basil. If you are trying to grow for the first time in a windowsill with moderate light, start with microgreens, lettuce, or spinach.

Make Sure to Try These *Growing Joy* Practices:

- Grow your own food (see page 74 for ideas if you are a beginner).
- Check out tips for growing tomatoes (see page 110).
- Try starting seeds (page 128). If you have started your own seeds already, I bet you'll be tickled by "The Show of Seed Starting" section (page 126).

Your Personality Will Shift and Change Just Like Your Plant Collection

It is totally normal to feel like a Mindful Plant Parent in one season of life and a Low-Key Plant Parent in another. It's likely that there is a little bit of every personality within your own, and the percentages fluctuate based on where you are in life. I like to say I'm 80 percent Mindful Plant Parent and 20 percent Low-Key Plant Parent.

These personality profiles are not meant to be the end-all-be-all, but rather a fun tool to dive deeper into your investigation of your plant/person relationship. Think about what resonated as you read this section and come back to it in a year to see if anything has shifted.

Know yourself, grow yourself, grow some joy, and don't take yourself too seriously.

Know Your Number

There is a very fine line between joyfully growing your plant collection and the tipping point many plant parents reach when their collections get too large and become a source of stress instead of joy. Finding the number of plants that brings delight instead of triggering anxiety is the key tip I can give you for growing joy. Everyone's "number" is different. One of my plant friends has six plants. She has a totally minimalist approach to her collection and revels in the simplicity and the intention behind each choice she's made in it. Her number is perfect for her. Another friend has more than three hundred plants and adores her plant care routine and the responsibilities that come with a collection that large. Her number is perfect for her.

Every plant parent's number is highly personal and will change as their lives change. Different homes and seasons of life will call for different numbers. The key is that your plant care routine and plant collection should help you relax and be a source of happiness (and, of course, allow you to keep yourself and your plants healthy and happy).

Tips for finding and maintaining your plant number

- Don't get attached to it. Understand that it will change in different seasons of life.
- Remember that your passion for collecting plants is a marathon, not a sprint.
- Take a quarterly or annual inventory of your plant collection and grade the level of joy each plant is bringing you. Would you like to spend a few more minutes caring for your plants, or would reclaiming some time from your plant care duties feel like a relief? If there is a plant

that has caused you more stress than joy in the last year, it might be time to rehome it with someone who is a perfect fit for it. Releasing plants that don't serve you is a great way to reinvest your time and energy into the plants that do work for your lifestyle.

- If you are struggling to curate your collection to work for you, consider giving yourself parameters to work within. Maybe you want to hone in on a specific genus of plant that you really enjoy. Maybe you want to stop adding plants to your collection, and focus on investing time and energy into how you can design with the plants you already have. Maybe you're bored with what you have and want to experiment with an entirely new type of plant or growing method to try and spark some new curiosity and excitement.

The Dark Side

"Grow Through What You Go Through"

I can't write a book about growing joy without acknowledging that sometimes, life is not joyful. There are seasons of life filled with immense loss, grief, and sadness that a houseplant can never heal. My hope is that in times when life is overwhelming and painful, you'll be able to find a moment of reprieve and peace with your plants by using some of these practices. There are also times when even our plant collections can become a source of stress, if not cultivated in a healthy, sustainable way. The chapter is dedicated to the undeniable dark moments we all face—on the large scale of our lives and on the small scale within our collections—and how to grow through them.

Find Your Light

Have you ever noticed that if you have a houseplant near a window, all of the leaves will turn and face the sun? That's phototropism, a plant's ability to find light by using the nifty hormone auxin to elongate cells within the plant to move the leaves to face the light source. Phototropism makes plants amazingly adaptable. It gives them a competitive edge. If a tomato plant is knocked on its side, the stem will literally hang a uey and grow toward the sun, even if that's at a right angle from how it was originally growing. It just thinks, "Oh, the sun's over there now? No problem— I'll move to make it work."

Surrounding ourselves with plants is not only important for the moments when we feel good, but also for the moments when we are feeling bad. They can remind us that growth is always happening, that dormancy is sometimes important, and that we are designed to do hard things, adapt, and evolve. They can serve as an external reflection of our internal world—a reminder to not only keep an eye on our collections for wilting, thirst, pests, or general unhappiness, but to watch our own hearts in the same way. They are our mirrors and greatest companions, who will sit with us, grow with us, wilt with us, and keep fighting—even when we all might be a little slower to face the sun.

Next time you are struggling, try using your green teachers to chase your blues away. Find a quiet moment with your plants and sit with yourself. Observe how your plant soaks in the sunlight. Turn inward and imagine you are a plant leaf, looking for the sun. Feel the sensation in your body of sorting through your darkness to find some light.

Dig Deep

Take out your journal and think about the following ideas:

- Find five things in your life you are currently excited about. If you can't think of anything, you can make it as simple as the dinner you want to make tonight or the new album from your favorite artist. The more you list, the more will come.

- Find areas of your life that you've been able to adapt in, like your plants do. When in your life have you found yourself in a new position or situation and managed to thrive? Trust that you can do so again.

- Where is there "light" in your life that you can lean toward? How can you orient your time and energy toward the good stuff?

- Trust that if you're in a season of darkness, it will pass and new growth will be on the way.

On Plant Death

At some point during your plant parenthood, one of your plants is going to die. Sweet plant friend, you are still worthy.

Plant death happens. It's truly part of the journey. For every beautifully curated Instagram photo filled with perfect-looking plants, there is a little houseplant graveyard of dead or struggling plants that didn't make the photo cut. Frankly, if you haven't lost a plant somewhere along your plant parenthood journey, you're probably not doing it right.

Although a plant's death can be an instrumental moment in helping you grow as a plant parent, plant death also makes many people fall out of love with the hobby and simply give up. It certainly happened to me in my plant-killer days. We've all been there: Your plant collection is thriving and growing, and you're filled with joy as you water your plants and admire their growth, feeling nothing but positive vibes in their presence. Then out of nowhere, boom! A succulent turns mushy, begonia leaves turn brown or yellow, or your fern simply drops dead. Your joy dies along with that poor plant.

Now, as you are shamefully burying your perished plant in your compost, backyard, or trash bin, you can't help but think, "I'm never going to get this right," or "All my plants are going to die," or "I'm a failure." You make it mean something about you as a person and a plant parent, and that "something" is usually extremely negative and unhelpful.

You are at an important crossroads, plant friend. You can choose to let this plant death empower you or defeat you. It's up to you; it's really that simple. You've got two options:

Option A: You let the plant death confirm your sneaking suspicion that you suck and will never

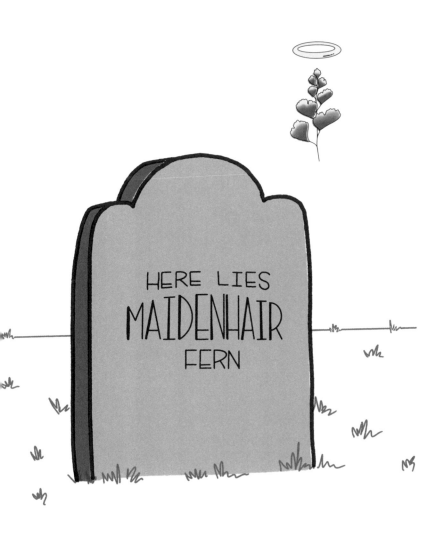

be good at anything, and you give up. You label yourself a "plant killer" and anecdotally joke about your plant fails while you admire someone's plant collection at a party and just stick with cut flowers in your home. I chose Option A for the first decade of adulthood. It sucked. I look back to those years and think about what my life might have been like if I had simply made the shift to option B earlier, and experienced the joy from plants that is so integral to my existence now. But enough about me.

Option B (hint . . . pick this one): You allow this plant death to make you curious and help you grow into a better plant parent. If something dies, ask yourself, "Hmm, what happened there?" Check the roots—did you accidentally overwater? Maybe you need to scale back your watering? Check the leaves for pests. Identify whatever little bugger wreaked havoc on your plant, research the shit out of it, and be prepared for next time. Maybe you realize that your plants don't thrive in a certain location, because you don't pass it often enough to remember to water the plants there? Maybe you become a better, wiser plant parent because of the lessons you learn and the research you do—all because of this one perished plant. Let's reframe plant deaths as a tremendously helpful part of plant care, instead of a failure.

On Plant Parent Overwhelm

We've talked a little bit about finding the right number of plants to have in your life and in your home. But what happens when we find ourselves on the wrong side of that line and our plant collections have become a burden in our lives instead of a blessing? I initially thought my struggles with plant parent overwhelm were unique, an outlier in our community, due to my dramatic and emotional tendencies. Then, I began to hear story after story from members of my listener community that bore an eerie resemblance to a period in my plant parent journey. I realized that Plant Parent Overwhelm is something we all struggle with.

When I started successfully caring for plants, after a few months there was a transition where I went from casually collecting plants to having plants take over most of the real estate in my brain. I was having so much fun with this new hobby that for a moment it felt like I couldn't stop. I was constantly thinking of plants, googling plants, buying new plants, and going to plant shops. It started to teeter on the verge of being unhealthy. I understand why people so often call someone a "Crazy Plant Lady." Once you start drinking the Plant Care Kool-Aid and your heart starts growing and opening up due to the success and beauty of your plant collection, it's easy to fall a little "crazy in love" with your new hobby.

Once every surface of our apartment was cluttered with plants, Billy actually had to have a little intervention to slow me down and make sure we had the space and knowledge to keep the plants healthy and to keep our home from looking like an episode of *Hoarders*. I've realized there is a fine line between "jungle vibes" and "hoarder nightmare." With his help (or maybe we should call it his gentle and loving insistence), I put myself on a plant pause that helped snap me out of that obsessive moment.

My story is not unique. Many people go through periods where they get a little "in over their skis" and need to "check themselves before they wreck themselves." It's part of the process.

If and when you ever find yourself in a moment of plant parent overwhelm, here are some tips:

- Accept that you are exactly where you need to be. This is a teachable moment in your plant parent journey, and you're doing great. Forgive yourself. This happens to everyone. It's *part* of being a plant parent. It's your next steps that will define how quickly you'll bounce back and create a healthy relationship with your new hobby.

- Assess where you are. What is currently causing you stress about your plants?

  - Has your collection gotten too large to manage? Consider gifting some plants to friends, or loaning plants to a plant friend to "babysit" until you can bring them back to your home with a more relaxed mindset.

- Are you unable to stop buying plants? Are you concerned about the sudden expense of your new purchasing habits? Put yourself on a plant pause and focus on your current collection. This will be hard at first, but it's SO worth it. See my "Tips for Going on a Plant Pause" below.

- Set a budget and stick to it! Spending over your budget is a key indicator that it might be time to take a deeper look at your approach to your plant collection.

- Find a focus. If your general plant collection is overwhelming you, consider niching down to a focus on a single type of plant. Get super curious about a certain genus of plants (*Peperomia*, *Dracaena*, and *Hoya* all have so many species you could deep-dive into), experiment with propagating, and spend time learning about the plants you already have.

- Work with what you've got. It's about quality, not quantity. When I took my plant pause, the first thing I did was organize all the plants I had in my collection. I'd been so focused on growing the collection, I hadn't even paid attention to styling or how the plants would fit in my home. I got a grow light to set up some high-light-loving plants for success. I organized plants on plant stands and shelves. I cleaned leaves and observed growth and tried to find moments of awe and joy in my current collection. There is so much you can do with a plant collection, without adding to it, so make a list of projects and get to work!

The Plant Pause

I think going on a plant pause is a really healthy practice for any plant parent, regardless of the size of the plant collection or the emotional state around it. Although collecting plants is super fun, pausing to assess how we can level up our current plant collection and drop into their needs is a great way to slow down, practice presence, and keep ourselves in check as our passion for plants grows.

Tips for going on a plant pause

- Define your rules. A plant pause can look different for different people. Here are some options:
    - Halt all spending on any aspect of plant care: plants, accessories, pots, lights—

the works. Really lean into what you already have, celebrate it, and cultivate it. Take this time to get to know the plants you already have.

- Stop bringing any plants (purchased or traded) home for a certain period of time.

- Assess your current "plant number" and decide if you need to reduce it by making plans to gift, donate, or sell your plants.

- Involve your community. Share your goals with whomever you live with and your closest friends. Billy asked me to go on a plant pause, so my situation is a bit unique. I was so out of control at that moment that I really needed an accountability partner to help me break the bad spending habits I was getting into. A positive side effect of this accountability was that once I started bringing plants home again, I would talk with him first, and our collection became more of a collaborative project. The pause ultimately brought us closer together and brought us more collective joy as a couple, because we both felt connected to the plants in our home on a deeper level.

- Set a time frame. Sometimes putting yourself on a plant pause with no end date can feel upsetting and unattainable. Setting a deadline helps. Anyone can stop buying plants for a month! For me, it was around six months (with several special exceptions) before I decided it was time to start adding to my collection again. Your pause could be as short as a week or as long as a year. But giving yourself those deadlines will provide you more freedom to really commit to it and actually enjoy the experience instead of resenting it.

- Be kind to yourself. We've all gotten into bad habits that need to be broken . . . and we all know how hard that can be. This might not be easy, and you might not be successful at first. Always keep in mind that you are trying to better yourself, and any step toward self-improvement is better than none.

- It's about quality, not quantity. Find your number and stick with it (until you can add or subtract from a healthy place). Focus on creating a thriving collection of happy plants that bring you joy. That truly can mean two plants for some people.

What to do while on a plant pause

- See how you can streamline and design the plant collection you currently have.

- Learn the Latin names of your plants.

- Learn to propagate your current plants.

- Take a deep dive into understanding the wild, complicated world of plant nutrition, and figure out your fertilizing plan.

- Repot and give the plants you have the TLC they need.

- Learn learn learn! Take a course at your local botanical garden, join my educational community, watch Plant Tube, binge podcasts, read blogs—expand your knowledge of plant care to help serve your collection and yourself.

A yoga teacher of mine once said, "The pose only begins when you start to get uncomfortable." That thought has stuck with me in my personal development journey. Sometimes growth happens when things start to itch. Pruning a plant back actually instigates new, bushier growth. Trees fall in the woods, and make space for new, younger saplings to grow into the canopy. An annual dies and decomposes to enrich the soil with more nutrients for new plants to thrive next year.

Overwhelm is okay. It's part of the process. It's how you respond to it that creates the good stuff. Use it as your teacher. Go back to the practices in this book to bring a smile to your face, and maybe even find deep joy in the process of working your way back.

11 Growing Together

When I think of growing joy, the first thing I think of is the happiness plants have brought *me*. This whole book is centered on using plants to increase our own happiness and mindful moments.

But here's the interesting thing . . . when I really drop in and think about growing joy, the warmest feelings come from remembering how these plants came into my home and *who* they came from. Many of my plants were tiny cuttings traded or gifted to me that have grown into large, luscious plants. Now they not only beautify my home, but also remind me of their stories. Yes: In addition to helping me disconnect from technology and reconnect with myself, the potted plants I love all hold stories that help me feel more connected to other plant parents, and the moments of generosity and kindness we shared because of them.

I acquired my first Swiss cheese plant (*M. deliciosa*) at a plant swap in exchange for a caladium (*Caladium* sp.). It was my number one wish-list plant; I was dying to have one of my own. Seeing it across the room at the plant swap was love at first sight. I remember the thrill of the thought of finally getting my hands on the plant I had seen in every magazine, figuring out how to strike up a conversation with its owner, and negotiating the trade. At the time of the swap, it was a cutting of a juvenile plant with unfenestrated leaves, meaning none of the leaves had the trademark holes that give the plant its famous silhouette. So much excitement and patience were focused on every new leaf over the next year, as I waited to see *if this would be the one* to unfurl with those famous windows in its leaves. The anticipation of watching the plant grow was as much fun as finally seeing it unfurl its first fenestrated leaf, and many more thereafter.

On my desk sits my first coin plant, or friendship plant (*P. peperomioides*). This plant is popular because of the little babies it grows, which are easy to separate and gift to friends; hence the name. When this plant was at peak popularity and was going for $40 for a small pot, I was fortunate enough to be gifted a plantlet by a friend I made online who turned into a true in-person friend.

My heirloom jade plant, which is over twenty years old, was gifted to me by a friend who unexpectedly had to move across the country. It's so large and has grown so much that I have since gifted several cuttings to my sister, who has then gifted cuttings to her friends. I love to think of the joy this single plant has brought to so many of us and how it honors the friend who had to part with it.

Making friends as an adult is hard, but making plant

MAKING FRIENDS AS AN ADULT IS HARD, BUT MAKING PLANT FRIENDS IS EASY

friends is easy, no matter what age you are. More often than not, you'll find that plant lovers are eager to share their knowledge and passion with others. When you meet another plant parent, you feel seen on a different level. The nurturer in you sees the nurturer in the other, and vice versa, and you both know you've found a safe place to nerd out, share your passion confidently, and learn from each other.

When I went from plant killer to plant lady, social media was the main way I was able to "meet" so many plant people around the world. I started connecting with people online, and once we developed a friendship, we organized safe ways to meet up in person to connect and deepen our relationship. Some of those friendships I made years ago are still going strong. Here are some tips for creating your own "plant friend posse" and growing a community of your own.

Virtually: Slide into the DMs of a Potential New Plant Friend

Okay, so we've established that plant parents are the kindest, coolest people, right? Have I mentioned they are also super friendly? The easiest way to start growing your community of plant friends is by doing what all the kids are doing these days—shoot them a message and strike up a conversation. Find fellow plant enthusiasts you admire, give them a follow on your social media of choice, and send them thoughtful messages about their plant collections. Mention you have the same plant and compare notes about your growing conditions. Compliments go a long way. In the beginning of your conversation, refrain from just messaging and asking for advice or free cuttings. Simply reach out, say hello, and go for an authentic connection. Let the conversation unfold organically.

I have a real love-hate relationship with social media, as authenticity is scarce and trolls are everywhere. But it has also been a beautiful instrument to foster genuine connections with people whom I would never have befriended and is an amazing way to connect with other plant enthusiasts. So give it a try, be kind, and have fun. If you're looking for a safe, fun online community of like-minded plant friends, check out the Bloom and Grow Garden Party Platform, detailed in the resource section at the end of this book.

Make #plantfriendsIRL

Before we dive into this section, I have to state the obvious: please do not put yourself in any type of dangerous situation when meeting new people. All of my in-person meetups with plant friends were always in public, in the middle of the day, surrounded by other people in public spaces. I always shared my location with Billy and never went back to anyone's home. Safety first, plant friends, safety first. Okay, back to our previously scheduled planty programming.

When I first started getting into plants, none of my friends were interested in hearing me talk about the magical scent of my tomato foliage. My friends knew me as a plant killer, and frankly, as plant killers themselves, they weren't interested in getting onboard with my new love. I felt a little lonely in my new passion. That's when I turned to Instagram, and with several searches for #houseplant, #plantparent, and #plantlover, my world was opened to the beautiful online community of plant lovers who were just like me. I started following people and accounts that resonated with me. After getting to know the collections, I messaged some of these people, and began to develop real relationships with them.

At the time I was living in NYC, which has a robust plant shop scene, and after vetting these virtual plant friends to make sure I wasn't getting catfished, I started making plans to meet in real life at plant shops. Plant shopping dates turned into lunch dates, which turned into dinners and genuine friendships. Our initial conversations around plant care evolved into regular conversations between two friends about normal life. Making adult friends can be hard, and plants were the entryway to genuine friendships that went beyond our shared hobby.

In addition to looking for like-minded plant friends online, be on the lookout for opportunities to connect with plant people "in the wild"—no screen required. I recently befriended a bartender at a local restaurant in my new neighborhood because of our shared plant love. Billy and I were there on a date, and my shirt had an illustration of the *P. peperomioides* on it, and she mentioned she had one. We got to chatting, and I told her how curious I was about *Hoya*, and, completely unprompted, she immediately offered me a cutting of her *Hoya carnosa* 'Krimson Princess'. That's a really "Happy Plant Lady" move, always looking to share the planty love with other plant people. We exchanged phone numbers and kept in touch about our planty projects that season and even exchanged plants. It was a sweet connection with a local in a new town I would have never made if it wasn't for the power of plants.

If you open your eyes to the concept of #plantfriends-IRL, you'll learn there are new friends to be made everywhere you turn.

Find Community: Organize a Plant Swap

If you've never been to a plant swap, you should try one. A plant swap can be as simple as an arrangement between two people who meet up and trade or as extensive as a citywide event with hundreds of people. Essentially, a plant swap is an event where plant parents come together with healthy, pest-free, rooted cuttings of their plants and trade with each other. They are an amazing way to meet other local plant parents and expand your collection for free. Plus it's fun to stay in touch with the people you swap with, and to follow how your gifted cutting is doing in its new home.

After I cultivated online friendships with a few members of the NYC plant community, several of us started a private message thread and named ourselves the NYC Plant Mamas. We hosted plant swaps and meetups in our homes across NYC and had fun afternoons trading, talking, laughing, and plant shopping together. These were private, free plant swaps that we created for ourselves. All it took was a teensy bit of organization and everyone being open to new friendships. But there are also ways to do this on a larger scale.

If messaging a stranger over social media is too much for you (which I totally get), connecting with your local plant shops and getting involved in community events is also a wonderful option. I took several plant care classes at local plant shops and attended a Homestead Brooklyn Plant Swap when I was first starting, and I am still friends with some of the people I met at those events years later. I want to recognize my dear plant friend Summer Rayne Oakes, of Homestead Brooklyn, who forever changed how plant swaps were done by leading the most epic citywide plant swaps in NYC. Summer Rayne and her YouTube channel, Homestead Brooklyn, are a great wealth of planty information. You can find more info on her in the "Resources" section of this book.

Plant shops are the hubs of local plant communities, so don't hesitate to call your local plant shops and see if they 1) have any swaps or events organized that you can attend or 2) would be interested in partnering with you to host a plant swap or event. If they don't already have organized events, plant swaps are a great way for them to bring new customers to their store; they already have the space and an email list of local clients to get some buzz going for the event. If you can't find a plant shop to host, you can also reach out to local bars, restaurants, and libraries, or to any social hub in your community.

I've hosted plant swaps ranging in size from two to fifty people. Here are some guidelines if you are interested in flexing your planty "hostess with the mostess" skills:

How to host a plant swap

- **Planning Phase**
  - Agree on a time, location, and max capacity for the event if you are meeting indoors.
  - Decide whether or not this will be entirely free or a paid event to cover costs.
  - Consider partnering with local vendors, like plant shops, restaurants, or stores that consider themselves community hubs, that might be able to offset rental costs for you in exchange for having their name attached to the event.
  - Figure out how you'll spread the word: research Facebook groups, reach out to

local plant people in your city, or get creative within your own social channels and community. If you're partnering with a plant shop, it might already have access to the plant community via an email list. In 2019, when I was traveling the country performing in the musical *Cats*, I reached out to local plant shops and plant friends I'd made on the internet to help me create live tapings of my podcasts and host listener meetups in local plant parent hubs. It was an amazing way to cultivate community.

- Create some sort of shareable photo or flyer about the swap with all of the information needed. Share with everyone you know! Canva.com has easy plug-and-play templates you can use for free.

- Plan your cuttings in advance and make several extra cuttings to bring to the swap in case someone hasn't gotten the chance to trade. You get to feel like Santa, spreading planty joy with surprise plant cuttings you gift to unsuspecting new plant friends.

- Order name tags! This was a huge lesson I learned through plant swaps and live events I've hosted for my podcast. Everyone should have a name tag with their name and social media handle. This will encourage people to follow each other and stay in touch, and is a lot less invasive than a phone number or email.

- Create a plant care card template everyone can fill out for their cuttings when they arrive at the swap. This can be as simple as small pieces of blank paper you instruct everyone to fill out with plant name and care, or you can get fancy and design a little card with the plant name, plant care suggestions, owner name, and social media handle, so people can stay in touch after they've swapped. I personally wish I'd taken better notes of whom I traded with at my first plant swaps, because I'd have loved to follow up with them and show them how large the cuttings they gave me have grown!

- Getting some light refreshments for the event is always a fun addition. You can pay for these out of pocket, use ticket sales to cover the cost, or ask the local business you are partnering with to provide them.

- **The Day Of**

  - Set up a table where everyone can put their plants and leave the plant care cards with instructions on how to fill them out and a box of pens or pencils.

  - Have the schedule of the day written somewhere where everyone can see. When people arrive, they should put their plants with the cards on the table and then mingle and see all the different plant options. I suggest letting everyone mingle for around twenty or thirty minutes to see the full selection (and to allow for latecomers) and then making a little speech to kick off the event. When I introduce an event, before the swapping begins, I like to ask everyone to turn to the person next to them, introduce themselves, and share their favorite plant. This is a nice, structured way for a roomful of strangers to break the ice before they start swapping.

  - It's a good idea to go over rules and remind everyone to relax and have fun.

Plant swaps can be nerve-racking for people, and the stakes can get a little high when rare plants are available. Remind everyone to keep it fair and kind.

- As the host, it's also your job to make sure no one leaves empty-handed. Some people will be shyer than others. Help people who are hovering on the outskirts of the swap by introducing them to others and helping them strike up their first conversations. Plant swapping can make people feel pretty vulnerable. At the root of it, you are offering something you love to see if someone is interested in it. That's not easy! When I went to my first plant swap, I was so intimidated by all the strangers and all the rare plants being traded that I almost left right then and there. As the host, although you'll likely be swapping yourself, keep an eye on the other swappers, and make sure to offer those extra cuttings you brought to those who haven't swapped yet.

- As the swap time is wrapping up, make sure to announce "closing time" so people know it's last call for swaps. Plants that have no takers can be put on the table as "up for grabs" for anyone who wants them. I've scored lots of plants by sticking around for the "up for grabs" portion of an event!

- Clean up: Make sure you have a cleanup plan with your cohosts. Ensure that the garbage gets taken out, the tables and floors get swept, and that you leave the space cleaner than it was when you arrived. Many people will offer to stay and help, so take them up on their offer and make sure you aren't leaving the generous local business that hosted you with hours of cleanup after you've left.

Garden with Different Generations: Connect with Your Elders and Youth

Although a lot of this chapter has to do with social media and the modern ways that members of our plant community find each other, there is truly nothing like connecting with a different generation of plant lovers off-line, whether it's helping young ones squeal in delight of watching seeds germinate and sprout roots, or soaking up the wisdom of our elders, who have decades of gardening experience under their belts to share with us. If you have children in your life, do germination experiments with them, help them set up their first herb garden, teach them how to grow strawberries, or give them their own special houseplant they get to care for on their own. I had a friend who built her daughter a fairy garden and used a small parlor palm (*Chamaedorea elegans*) as the backdrop! Keep the plant community thriving for the generations to come by getting our future generations excited about plants and growing their own food from a young age. It will light you up like a full-spectrum grow light.

No amount of googling is going to beat fifty years of gardening experience. Some of my most fun plant friendships are with seniors who have been gardening for decades and who are ready to plant seeds of knowledge in younger generations. Taking time to make friends the old-fashioned way, by actually joining a local garden club and engaging with elders of your community, is a beautiful way to learn lessons a book can never teach you.

When I first moved from five hundred square feet in NYC to five acres in the woods, I was itching to garden outdoors. I had never had land, and was filled with the desire to grow my own food, and to take my relationship with plants and nature to the next level. But here's the thing: There are deer in the woods. And bears. And ticks and chipmunks and moles and voles, and this city girl was *way* out of her element.